WK 12   R2-

Baillière's
CLINICAL
GASTROENTEROLOGY
INTERNATIONAL PRACTICE AND RESEARCH

Baillière's

CLINICAL

GASTROENTEROLOGY

INTERNATIONAL PRACTICE AND RESEARCH

Volume 10/Number 3
September 1996

Liver and Gastrointestinal Immunology

M. P. MANNS MD
Guest Editor

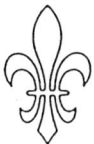

Baillière Tindall
London Philadelphia Sydney Tokyo Toronto

This book is printed on acid-free paper.

Baillière Tindall
W.B. Saunders
Company Ltd

24–28 Oval Road
London NW1 7DX, UK

The Curtis Center, Independence Square West,
Philadelphia, PA 19106–3399, USA

55 Horner Avenue
Toronto, Ontario M8Z 4X6, Canada

Harcourt Brace & Company
Australia
30–52 Smidmore Street, Marrickville, NSW 2204, Australia

Harcourt Brace & Company
Japan Inc
Ichibancho Central Building,
22–1 Ichibancho, Chiyoda-ku, Tokyo 102, Japan

Whilst great care has been taken to maintain the accuracy of the information contained in this issue, the authors, editor, owners and publishers cannot accept any responsibility for any loss or damage arising from actions or decisions based on information contained in this publication; ultimate responsibility for the treatment of patients and interpretation of published material lies with the medical practitioner. The opinions expressed are those of the authors and the inclusion in this publication of material relating to a particular product, method or technique does not amount to an endorsement of its value or quality, or of the claims made by its manufacturer.

ISSN 0950–3528

ISBN 0–7020–2187–3 (single copy)

Baillière's Clinical Gastroenterology is published four times each year by Baillière Tindall. Prices for Volume 10 (1996) are:

TERRITORY	ANNUAL SUBSCRIPTION	SINGLE ISSUE
Europe including UK	£102.00 (Institutional) post free	£30.00 post free
	£87.00 (Individual) post free	
All other countries	Consult your local Harcourt Brace & Company office	

The editor of this publication is Ian Bramley, Baillière Tindall, 24–28 Oval Road, London NW1 7DX, UK.

Baillière's Clinical Gastroenterology is covered in Index Medicus, Current Contents/Clinical Medicine, Current Contents/Life Sciences, the Science Citation Index, SciSearch, Research Alert and Excerpta Medica.

Baillière's Clinical Gastroenterology was published from 1972 to 1986 as *Clinics in Gastroenterology*

Typeset by Phoenix Photosetting, Chatham.
Printed and bound in Great Britain by the University Printing House, Cambridge, UK.

Contributors to this issue

STEPHAN C. BISCHOFF MD, Division of Gastroenterology and Hepatology, Medical School of Hannover, Konstanty-Gutschow Strasse 8, D-30623 Hannover, Germany.

PETER T. DONALDSON BSc, PhD, Head of Immunogenetics, Institute of Liver Studies, King's College Hospital, Denmark Hill, London SE5 9RS, UK.

CLAUDIO GALPERIN MD, Research Specialist, Division of Rheumatology, Allergy and Clinical Immunology, TB 192, University of California Davis School of Medicine, Davis, CA 95616, USA.

M. ERIC GERSHWIN MD, Professor of Medicine; Chief of Rheumatology, Division of Rheumatology, Allergy and Clinical Immunology, TB 192, University of California, Davis School of Medicine, Davis, CA 95616, USA.

MICHAEL GÖKE MD, Research Fellow, Gastrointestinal Unit, Massachusetts General Hospital, Harvard Medical School, 32 Fruit Street, Boston, MA 02114, USA.

GEORG KÖHNE MD, Department of Internal Medicine II, University of Saarland, D-66421 Homburg/Saar, Germany.

MICHAEL P. MANNS MD, Professor of Medicine; Director, Division of Gastroenterology and Hepatology, Medical School of Hannover, Konstanty-Gutschow Strasse 8, D-30623 Hannover, Germany.

LLOYD MAYER MD, Professor of Medicine & Microbiology; Chief, Division of Clinical Immunology, Mount Sinai Hospital, One Gustave L. Levy Place, Box 1089, NY 10029, USA.

PETRA OBERMAYER-STRAUB PhD, Senior Research Associate, Division of Gastroenterology and Hepatology, Medical School of Hannover, Konstanty-Gutschow Strasse 8, D-30623 Hannover, Germany.

ASIT PANJA MD, Assistant Professor of Medicine, Mount Sinai Hospital, One Gustave L. Levy Place, Box 1089, NY 10029, USA.

DANIEL K. PODOLSKY MD, Gastrointestinal Unit, GRJ-719, Massachusetts General Hospital, Harvard Medical School, 50 Fruit Street, Boston, MA 02114, USA.

BARBARA REHERMANN MD, Division of Gastroenterology and Hepatology, Medical School of Hannover, Konstanty-Gutschow Strasse 8, D-30623 Hannover, Germany.

THOMAS SCHNEIDER PhD, MD, Department of Internal Medicine II, University of Saarland, D-66421 Homburg/Saar, Germany.

MARTIN ZEITZ MD, Director, Professor of Medicine, Department of Internal Medicine II, University of Saarland, D-66421 Homburg/Saar, Germany.

Table of contents

PREVIOUS ISSUES

FORTHCOMING ISSUE

Preface

One of the body's most important 'organs' is the immune system, with its ability to protect the body from attack by various pathogenic agents, e.g. viruses, bacteria, fungi and parasites. To do this the immune system has to distinguish between self and non-self, which can only be achieved by sophisticated regulatory systems. Misregulations in these complex functions will adversely affect individual organs or be the cause of systemic auto-immune diseases. A main access for invasive pathogenic agents is the gastrointestinal tract which contains the majority of the body's immune system amounting to approximately two-thirds of the overall number of immune cells. Thus it stands to reason that a number of diseases are mediated by a pathological reaction of the mucosal immune system, presumably such immune-mediated diseases as ulcerative colitis and Crohn's disease. Also of clinical importance is mucosal allergy.

The authors included here have contributed to *Baillière's Clinical Gastroenterology* in an attempt to provide a comprehensive update on the physiology of the mucosal immune system. This issue includes chapters by Panja and Mayer, dealing with antigen presentation in the intestine, Köhne, Schneider and Zeitz on the special features of the intestinal lymphocytic system compared to other parts of the immune system and Göke and Podolsky who provide us with important information on the regulation of the mucosal epithelial barrier. Of increasing clinical importance are the mechanisms of mucosal allergy with food allergy presenting a huge problem. As the gastrointestinal tract presents the largest surface of the body, one wonders why mucosal allergy (as discussed by Bischoff) in clinical medicine is frequently underestimated when compared to allergies of the skin and the respiratory tract.

The immune system is also involved in the pathophysiology of many diseases of the liver. Five major hepatitis viruses have been characterized and the hepatitis G/GB viruses have recently been discovered. It is obvious that for all these viruses the host's immune system is crucial for the manifestation and the clinical course of the disease. Rehermann concentrates on the current and steadily increasing knowledge of cellular immune reactions against particular antigens of the major hepatitis viruses. This new information on the mechanisms of T cell immunology against hepatitis viruses may lead to new therapeutic strategies including T cell vaccination. A further increasingly important issue in hepatology are autoimmune liver diseases. Calperin and Gershwin provide an overview on the immuno-pathology of primary biliary cirrhosis, a disease regarded as an auto-immune reaction against bile duct epithelium. Less than 10 years ago the molecular identity of mitochondrial antigens was discovered. Now important groups, like that of Gershwin, are struggling to use this knowledge to unravel the aetiology and pathogenesis of this disease. In autoimmune hepatitis the autoimmune reaction is directed against the major liver cell, the hepatocyte. Cytochrome P450 enzymes and members of the UDP-glucuronosyltransferases have been identified as autoantigens in genuine autoimmune hepatitis and in some patients with viral hepatitis. To date it is unknown whether the fact that specific microsomal auto-antibodies are present in patients with viral hepatitis, has an impact on the immunopathogenesis of these viral diseases. Finally, a minority of adverse drug reactions are immune-mediated and in some of these cases specific autoimmunity against drug-metabolizing enzymes is observed. Obermayer-Straub and myself present current thinking on the molecular character-ization of microsomal target antigens in autoimmune hepatitis, viral hepatitis, hepatitis as component in autoimmune polyendocrine syndrome 1, and drug-induced liver disease. Finally, it is indisputable that immuno-genetics are of particular relevance in the pathophysiology of viral and autoimmune liver diseases. Donaldson provides an overview on the present knowledge of the immunogenetics of autoimmune liver disease, in particu-lar primary biliary cirrhosis, autoimmune hepatitis and primary sclerosing cholangitis. This knowledge certainly increases our understanding of the mechanisms leading to liver tissue destruction in viral and autoimmune liver disease.

M. P. MANNS

1

Regulation of the mucosal epithelial barrier

MICHAEL GÖKE
DANIEL K. PODOLSKY

The intestinal epithelial monolayer forms a barrier which interfaces with a complex external milieu including microorganisms, antigens, dietary substances, and a mixture of host digestive enzymes. The epithelial surface of the intestinal tract comprises various epithelial populations, including primarily columnar cells (enterocytes and colonocytes) and goblet cells as well as the less abundant entero-endocrine and Paneth cell populations in addition to more minor cell populations (e.g. tuft cells). The mucosal surface of the intestinal tract is virtually unique in the rapid and continued turnover of the mucosal surface throughout life. Indeed, the epithelial surface of the small and large intestine exhibits the most rapid constitutive cell turnover in the body, occurring every 24–96 hours in man and other mammalian species (Lipkin et al, 1963). Thus it must maintain an exquisite balance between proliferation and cell loss while preserving the structural continuity and functional integrity of the epithelial cell surface.

Rapid re-sealing of the epithelial barrier is necessary after any form of injury, for example, mucosal erosions or ulcerations due to peptic lesions, inflammatory bowel disease, infectious agents and/or their toxins, ischaemia or radiation. Repair of epithelial lesions in the gastrointestinal tract has been shown to involve at least two distinct processes. First, viable epithelial cells migrate from areas adjacent to the injured surface to cover the denuded area. This process, which has been observed in vivo and in vitro, has been termed restitution (Rutten and Ito, 1983; Silen, 1987; Feil et al 1987; Lacy 1988; Waller et al, 1988; Feil et al, 1989a,b; Moore et al, 1989; McCormack et al, 1992; Nusrat et al, 1992). In vivo, restitution appears to be an initial mechanism to prevent deeper mucosal damage. Restitution can re-establish epithelial continuity within minutes to hours, a much shorter time-frame than that needed for cell proliferation. Following re-establishment of surface epithelial continuity, cell proliferation enables replacement of lost epithelial cell populations. The latter process is thought to begin 12–16 hours after injury and takes one to several days to complete.

While cell proliferation of intestinal epithelial cells has been studied intensively, much less is known about the process of restitution. Recent work has demonstrated that various peptide growth factors present in the intestinal mucosa modulate intestinal epithelial cell proliferation.

Baillière's Clinical Gastroenterology—
Vol. 10, No. 3, September 1996
ISBN 0–7020–2187–3
0950–3528/96/030393 + 13 $12.00/00

Extracellular matrix molecules of the basement membrane/lamina propria produced by both epithelial and lamina propria cell populations (most notably pericryptal fibroblasts) have also been shown to modulate intestinal epithelial cell growth. In addition, the trefoil family of peptides, goblet cell products that are secreted onto the luminal surface, also appear to be functionally important for the preservation of intestinal epithelial integrity.

Epithelial cells that line the intestinal tract act as absorptive and secretory cells. The concept that intestinal epithelial cells function exclusively in nutrient absorption, electrolyte transport, and mucin glycoprotein production and secretion has been challenged by recent findings demonstrating that intestinal epithelial cells can also express cytokines and cytokine receptors known to be important in the communication between inflammatory cells and cells of the immune system. These observations, together with reports that human intestinal epithelial cells are able to take up, process and present soluble antigens in vitro (Mayer and Shlien, 1987) and express MHC class II molecules in vitro and in vivo (Scott et al, 1980, Selby et al, 1983; Mayer et al, 1991) suggest an unanticipated additional role of intestinal epithelial cells as a component of host mucosal immune response.

This article focuses on recent advances in the understanding of the functional role of the complex network of mucosal cytokines, extracellular matrix molecules, and trefoil peptides in intestinal epithelial barrier function. These factors appear to be physiologically important for the maintenance of intestinal epithelial continuity and they substantially modulate intestinal epithelial restitution in the initial response to superficial mucosal lesions after injury.

THE ROLE OF MUCOSAL CYTOKINES IN MUCOSAL INTEGRITY

The peptide growth factors TGF-α and TGF-β have both been shown to be expressed in intestinal epithelial cells and appear to be important modulators of intestinal epithelial cell growth (Kurokawa et al, 1987; Koyama and Podolsky, 1989; Suemori et al, 1991a; Podolsky and Babyatsky, 1995). Transforming growth factor (TGF)-α is a strong promoter and TGF-β1 a potent inhibitor of intestinal epithelial cell proliferation. Insulin-like growth factor (IGF)-I and -II, hepatocyte growth factor (HGF) and members of the fibroblast growth factor (FGF) family, including acidic and basic FGF and keratinocyte growth factor (KGF) increase intestinal epithelial cell proliferation in vitro and in vivo (Dignass et al, 1994a,c; Housley et al, 1994; Potten et al, 1995; Steeb et al, 1995).

While it was known that inhibition of polyamine synthesis and acidic pH decrease restitution (Feil et al, 1989a; McCormack et al, 1992) little was known about the effects of peptide growth factors. An in vitro model of intestinal epithelial restitution (McCormack et al, 1992; Ciacci et al, 1993a) using wounded confluent monolayers of non-transformed rat small intestinal epithelial crypt cells (IEC-6, Quaroni et al, 1979) has been a useful model for the study of early re-epithelialization after injury. In this model TGF-β1 was found to promote intestinal epithelial cell migration (Ciacci et al, 1993a). Addition of immunoneutralizing anti-TGF-β antibodies to otherwise untreated wounded monolayers was observed to suppress the baseline migration, suggesting that TGF-β is indeed a key endogenous product of this epithelial population promoting cell migration from the wound edge.

Various other regulatory peptides/cytokines present in the intestinal mucosa also modulate epithelial cell migration. TGF-α, epidermal growth factor (EGF), interleukin (IL)-1β, and interferon (IFN)-γ enhanced epithelial restitution by 2.3- to 5.5-fold (Dignass and Podolsky, 1993) and increased production of bioactive TGF-β1 peptide in wounded IEC-6 cell monolayers. In contrast, IL-6, tumour necrosis factor-α (TNF-α), platelet-derived growth factor (PDGF), and the endotoxin lipopolysaccharide (LPS) were not found to have a significant effect on intestinal epithelial cell migration. The promotion of IEC-6 cell restitution by TGF-α, EGF, IL-1β and IFN-γ could also be completely abrogated by the addition of immunoneutralizing anti-TGF-β1 antibodies, suggesting that these effects are mediated through a TGF-β1-dependent pathway by increasing the cellular production and secretion of bio-active TGF-β1. The importance of TGF-β1 was supported by recent confirmatory observations that TGF-β1 also enhanced intestinal epithelial barrier function in a T-84 cell model as reflected by an increase of electrical transepithelial resistance and decreased macromolecule permeability (Planchon et al, 1994).

Several other peptide growth factors have also been found to promote restitution in vitro. Basic FGF, KGF and HGF all enhanced migration of wounded IEC-6 cell monolayers (Dignass et al, 1994a,c). The enhancement of restitution was independent of cell proliferation. In vitro studies using the T-84 cell model confirmed that HGF increases restitution (Nusrat et al, 1994). In other studies basic FGF was observed to facilitate rapid epithelial repair of frog gastric mucosa in Ussing chamber experiments (Paimela et al, 1993).

It has also been found that IEC-6 cells as well as primary rat enterocytes express functional IL-2 receptors which respond to IL-2 stimulation with an initial increase in cell proliferation followed by inhibition (Ciacci et al, 1993b). Subsequent studies demonstrated the expression of the IL-2 receptor β chain and common γ (γc) chain in human colonic epithelial cells by reverse-transcription polymerase chain reaction (Reinecker and Podolsky, 1995). It was also shown that primary human colonic epithelial cells express transcripts for IL-4, IL-7 and IL-9 receptors. These receptors are remarkable for their shared utilization of the γc receptor chain of the IL-2 receptor. Receptors for IL-2, IL-4, IL-7 and IL-9 on intestinal epithelial cells appear to be functional as demonstrated by rapid tyrosine phosphorylation of proteins upon stimulation with the corresponding cytokines. These data are consistent with findings that the addition of IL-4 to intestinal epithelial cells (confluent T-84 cell monolayers) leads to significant reduction in transepithelial resistance (up to 70%) in a dose- and time-dependent manner that can be inhibited by neutralizing anti-IL-4 receptor antibodies (Colgan et al, 1994). Additionally, intestinal epithelial cells have also been shown to express transcripts for chemokines such as monocyte-chemoattractant protein-1 (MCP-1) and IL-8 (Eckmann et al, 1993, Jung et al, 1995). In summary, these data support the concept that intestinal epithelial cells, in addition to their capacity to absorb nutrients, transport electrolytes, and secrete components of the mucous layer, may also interact with immune and inflammatory cells within the intestinal mucosa and therefore are an integrated part of the mucosal immune system. Although the full functional role of epithelial cells in the immune response remains to be defined, these molecules may be involved in restitution through modulation of bio-active TGF-β.

THE ROLE OF EXTRACELLULAR MATRIX/BASEMENT MEMBRANE MOLECULES IN MUCOSAL INTEGRITY

The understanding of interactions between intestinal epithelial cells and the underlying extracellular matrix in intestinal epithelial restitution is still incomplete. The intestinal epithelial cell layer resides on a basement membrane which serves as the interface with the lamina propria. Basement membranes are composed predominantly of laminin, type IV collagen, nidogen/ entactin, and heparan sulphate proteoglycans (Timpl and Dziadek, 1986). Fibronectin has also been found in the basement membrane of the intestine (Laurie et al, 1982, Quaroni et al, 1978). Small amounts of fibronectin have been documented in adult intestinal basement membranes underlying villi (Laurie et al, 1982, Quaroni et al, 1978) and prominent expression has been found in basement membranes of crypts (Quaroni et al, 1978). Recent studies in this laboratory showed that non-transformed rat intestinal crypt epithelial cells express fibronectin, laminin β1 and laminin γ1 (according to new laminin nomenclature: Burgeson et al, 1994) transcripts and protein as well as low levels of collagen IV ($\alpha1/\alpha2$) but not laminin $\alpha1$ (Göke et al, 1996). These observations, in context with the distinct spatial expression pattern in the intestinal basement membrane along the crypt–villus axis suggest that fibronectin may be a structural component of basement membranes in the crypts of Lieberkühn, synthesized and deposited, at least in part, by intestinal epithelial cells. Although mesenchymal cells are thought to be the principal source of basement membrane collagen IV (Simon-Assmann et al, 1990; Weiser et al, 1990) studies utilizing IEC-6 cells support observations that small intestinal crypt cells may contribute to the synthesis of intestinal basement membrane collagen IV (Hahn et al, 1987). A lack of laminin $\alpha1$ transcripts and protein expression in IEC-6 cells—in contrast to laminin β1 and γ1—might be explained by the possible necessity of mesenchymal–epithelial interactions for expression of laminin $\alpha1$ and its deposition in intestinal basement membranes. Epithelial–mesenchymal interactions are thought to be critical for the formation of a complete basement membrane in the intestine (Hahn et al, 1987; Weiser et al, 1990; Simo et al, 1992b). IEC-6 cells might also express alternatives to the classic laminin $\alpha1$ chain, for example the laminin $\alpha 2$ chain of merosin or the $\alpha 3$ chain of kalinin/nicein, k-laminin, and ks-laminin (Ehrig et al, 1990; Marinkowich et al, 1992; Burgeson et al, 1994; Gerecke et al, 1994; Vuolteenaho et al, 1994). Interestingly, in the human small intestine, laminin $\alpha 1$ expression is restricted to the basement membrane of the villus while laminin $\alpha 2$ is found in the crypt basement membrane (Beaulieu and Vachon, 1994; Simon-Assmann et al, 1994). The functional importance of these observed laminin α chain expression patterns remains to be elucidated.

It is well recognized that the extracellular matrix on which epithelial cells reside modulates intestinal epithelial cell adhesion, morphogenesis and differentiation (Carroll et al, 1988; Hahn et al, 1990; Olson et al, 1991; Simo et al, 1992a; Moore et al, 1994; Turowski et al, 1994; Vachon and Beaulieu, 1995). Basement membrane turnover studies indicate that intestinal epithelial cells migrate over the basement membrane and that a synchronous migration of epithelial cells and the underlying basement membrane as a unit from crypt to villus tip does not occur (Trier et al, 1990). However, little is known about the functional role of the extra-cellular matrix in intestinal epithelial restitution in vivo.

Migration studies in wounded IEC-6 cell monolayers have shown that peptides which specifically compete with the major cell attachment site on fibronectin strongly inhibit cell migration in the restitution phase after epithelial wounding. A spatial expression pattern of fibronectin in intestinal basement membranes along the crypt–villus axis with prominent expression only in the crypt may explain observations in models utilizing CaCo-2 cells (but not the non-transformed, undifferentiated crypt epithelial cell line IEC-6) in which fibronectin did not appear to stimulate cell migration (Basson et al, 1992). However, the observation that fibronectin appears to promote migration of simple columnar epithelial cells such as intestinal crypt epithelial cells is consistent with effects of fibronectin in stratified epithelial populations, including wounded corneal epithelial cells (Nishida et al, 1983) and keratinocytes (O'Keefe et al, 1985; Sarret et al, 1992) in vitro.

It has also been suggested that collagen types III and IV modulate intestinal epithelial restitution in an in vitro guinea-pig model as demonstrated by the inhibition of restitution in the presence of both anti-collagen III and IV antibodies (Moore et al, 1992). Collagen type IV function-inhibiting antibodies directed against the main non-collagenous domain (NC1) at the carboxy-terminal part of the molecule also substantially impaired IEC-6 cell migration. In contrast, neutralizing anti-laminin anti-sera had no significant effect on restitution (Göke et al, 1996). These function-blocking studies are consistent with migration experiments using cell culture dishes pre-coated with fibronectin, type IV collagen, or laminin ($\alpha 1/\beta 1/\gamma 1$). Collectively, these observations support the concept that fibronectin and type IV collagen but not laminin enhance intestinal crypt epithelial cell restitution.

In the context of the apparent importance of some extracellular matrix components in restitution, it is noteworthy that TGF-$\beta 1$ up-regulates extra-cellular matrix molecule mRNA and protein expression by wounded IEC-6 cells compared with untreated wounded intestinal epithelial cells. This observation, in conjunction with the previous findings that TGF-β1 promotes, and immunoneutralizing anti-TGF-β antibodies inhibit, intestinal epithelial restitution, indicates that this growth factor may mediate its restitution-enhancing effects, at least in part, through modulation of expression of fibronectin and collagen type IV and perhaps other extracellular matrix components in intestinal epithelial cells. Although laminin (α1/β1/γ1) appears not to play a role in restitution, it may contribute to other processes involved in tissue repair, for example, differentiation and organization of intestinal epithelial cells as reported for model small intestinal and colonic epithelial cell lines (IEC-6, CaCo-2) as well as fetal intestinal epithelial cells in vitro (Carroll et al, 1988; Hahn et al, 1990; Olson et al, 1991; Vachon and Beaulieu, 1995). Interestingly, synthetic laminin peptides have also been found to stimulate neutrophil motility (Harvath et al, 1994).

The functional role of other components of the intestinal basement membrane, for example, entactin/nidogen and heparan sulphate, for intestinal epithelial restitution is largely unknown and will need to be defined by future studies. The reports that the heparan proteoglycan sulphate molecule perlecan is a potent inducer of high-affinity binding of basic FGF to its receptor and a promoter of basic FGF bio-activities (Burgess and Maciag 1989; Ruoslahti and Yamaguchi, 1991; Yayon et al, 1991; Aviezer et al, 1994) adds another potential role for extracellular matrix/basement membrane molecules in mucosal physiology and pathophysiology. It is likely that extracellular matrix molecules are not only structural proteins, but are also able to modulate fundamental intestinal epithelial functions important for mucosal barrier function.

THE ROLE OF TREFOIL PROTEINS AND MUCIN GLYCOPROTEINS IN MUCOSAL INTEGRITY

Although the epithelial monolayer represents the cellular surface of the intestinal mucosa, it has long been appreciated that the apical surface of this population is covered by a visco-elastic layer which comprises the interface between the lumen and the mucosa. This overlying coat consists largely of secreted products of the goblet cell population. Among these, the high-molecular-weight glycoproteins are the best known. Although these heterogeneous, highly glycosylated glycoproteins presumably contribute to the formation of a viscous gel layer, their functional role for mucosal integrity is still incompletely understood. Over recent years it has become clear that mucus-producing cells also secrete large amounts of trefoil peptides onto the luminal surface. The mammalian trefoil family of peptides encompasses at least three peptides (pS2, HSP and ITF) sharing a distinctive motif of six cysteine residues (designated trefoil or 'P' domain) which leads to the formation of three intrachain loops through disulphide bonding (Thim, 1988, 1989). Trefoil peptides are expressed in an organ-specific pattern throughout the gastrointestinal tract. pS2 expression is found in the proximal stomach and human spasmolytic polypeptide (HSP) in the distal stomach and biliary tree (and also pancreas in some species). Intestinal trefoil factor (ITF) has been detected throughout the small and large intestine (Jørgensen et al, 1982; Rio et al, 1988; Tomasetto et al, 1990; Suemori et al, 1991b; Chinery et al, 1992; Hanby et al, 1993; Podolsky et al, 1993; Jeffrey et al, 1994; Mashimo et al, 1995).

The presence of both trefoil peptides and mucin glycoproteins overlying the mucosal surface of the normal gastrointestinal tract suggests that these might play a role in sustaining integrity of the mucosal barrier. Studies have demonstrated that various trefoil peptides enhance migration of IEC-6 cells (3–6-fold) to re-establish continuity of wounded confluent monolayers. Trefoil factors promote restitution in a synergistic fashion (up to 15-fold) with mucin glycoproteins (Dignass et al, 1994b). However, trefoil factors do not appear to have a significant effect on proliferation of any of several transformed and non-transformed cell lines derived from human or rat gastrointestinal epithelium. In contrast to cytokine-mediated stimulation of intestinal epithelial cell restitution described above, trefoil peptide and combined trefoil peptide–mucin glycoprotein stimulation of intestinal epithelial restitution is not associated with significant changes in the production of bio-active TGF-β1 and is not affected by function-blocking anti-TGF-β antibodies. This indicates that trefoil factors found at the apical surface of the gastrointestinal tract exert their effects through a pathway distinct from that used by cytokines, which may act at the basolateral cell surface of the epithelial monolayer.

In other series of experiments, the effects of trefoil factors on intestinal epithelial barrier function have been characterized (Kindon et al, 1995). In these studies, T-84 cells which form tight polarized monolayers—and therefore a relatively impermeable barrier to the inert marker ^{3}H mannitol when grown on a transwell membrane support—were used as an intestinal epithelial model cell line. The addition of physiological doses of trefoil factors alone resulted in up to 50% attenuation of damage to monolayer integrity as measured by the decrease of ^{3}H-labelled mannitol penetration after various forms of epithelial injury (phytohemagglutinin, bile salts, oleic acid and taurocholic acid, or *Clostridium difficile* toxin A). Protection as much as 95% was achieved by the concomitant presence of colonic mucin glycoproteins. In contrast, non-mucin glycoproteins alone or in combination with trefoil peptides did not protect against injury. Collectively, these studies support the hypothesis that trefoil peptides and mucin glycoproteins interact in a synergistic manner and are important molecules for preserving mucosal integrity under normal circumstances as well as after various forms of intestinal epithelial injury.

In recent studies, it was demonstrated that trefoil peptides exert mucosal protective effects in vivo (Babyatsky et al, 1996). Oral recombinant HSP and ITF markedly protected against both ethanol and indomethacin-induced gastric injury in rats when given up to 6 hours before injury. These effects were not mediated by change of gastric pH and were also not associated with systemic absorption of trefoil factors. These observations support the conclusion that the visco-elastic gel layer formed by these

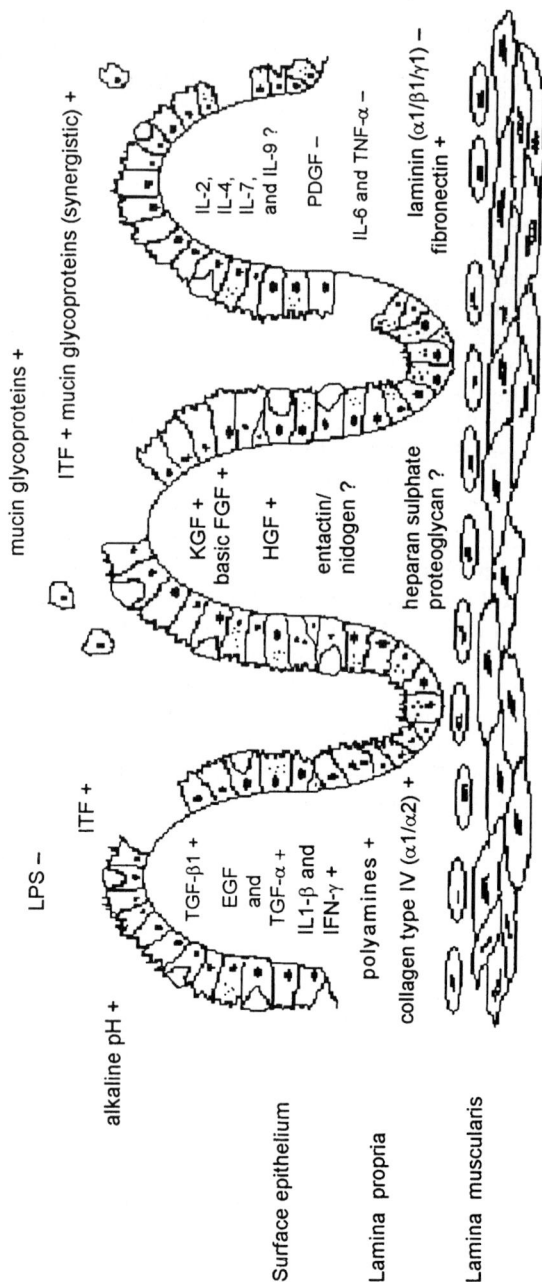

mucin glycoproteins +

ITF + mucin glycoproteins (synergistic) +

IL-2,
IL-4,
IL-7,
and IL-9 ?

PDGF –

IL-6 and TNF-α –

laminin (α1/β1/γ1) –
fibronectin +

LPS –

ITF +

KGF +
basic FGF +

HGF +

entactin/
nidogen ?

heparan sulphate
proteoglycan ?

alkaline pH +

TGF-β1 +

EGF
and
TGF-α +

IL1-β and
IFN-γ +

polyamines +

collagen type IV (α1/α2) +

Surface epithelium

Lamina propria

Lamina muscularis

Figure 1. Schematic illustration of the epithelium of the (small) intestinal mucosa including a denuded area. Apically and basolaterally acting factors (abbreviated as explained in the text) and their effects on intestinal epithelial restitution are shown. Symbols: + = increases restitution, − = no effect on restitution, ? = effect on restitution not defined.

constituents provides an important defence mechanism for protection of the mucosa from injury as well as facilitating repair after epithelial injury has occurred. The physiological relevance of trefoil peptides for mucosal repair is supported by the finding of increased or ectopic trefoil factor expression in close proximity to gastrointestinal ulceration (Wright et al, 1990; Rio et al, 1991; Wright et al, 1993; Taupin et al, 1994a,b, Cook et al, 1995; Stettler et al, 1995).

SUMMARY

Rapid re-sealing of the intestinal epithelial barrier is initially accomplished by migration of viable epithelial cells from the wound edge into the denuded area ('restitution') and only later by cell proliferation. Whereas proliferation of intestinal epithelial cells has been studied intensively, much less is known about the pivotal initial phase of cell migration. Restitution appears to be modulated by peptide growth factors/cytokines, extracellular matrix molecules, and luminally secreted products of mucus-producing cells (schematically summarized in Figure 1). Recent work has demonstrated that various cytokines (TGF-β1, TGF-α, EGF, IL-1β, IFN-γ, basic FGF, KGF and HGF) present in the intestinal mucosa enhance intestinal epithelial restitution, presumably by mediating its effects through the basolateral pole of the epithelial monolayer. In addition to their effects on cell adhesion, differentiation, and spatial organization, the extracellular matrix molecules on which intestinal epithelial cells reside also have the potential to stimulate intestinal epithelial cell migration. The basement membrane components fibronectin and collagen type IV may be especially important. Finally, trefoil factors, a recently identified family of peptides which are secreted onto the luminal surface where they form the visco-elastic mucus layer through interaction with mucin glycoproteins, also promote the important process of restitution through a pathway distinct from that used by factors acting at the basolateral cell surface.

Acknowledgements

Cited studies which were carried out in Dr D. K. Podolsky's laboratory were supported by grants from the National Institutes of Health (DK41557, DK43351 and DK46768 to D.K.P.). M.G. is a recipient of a postdoctoral fellowship grant from the Else Kröner-Fresenius-Stiftung.

REFERENCES

Aviezer D, Hecht D, Safran M et al (1994) Perlecan, basal lamina proteoglycan, promotes basic fibroblast growth factor-receptor binding, mitogenesis, and angiogenesis. *Cell* **79:** 1005–1013.
Babyatsky MW, DeBeaumont M, Thim L & Podolsky DK (1996) Oral trefoil peptides protect against ethanol- and indomethacin-induced gastric injury in rats. *Gastroenterology* **110:** 489–497.
Basson MD, Modlin IM & Madri JA (1992) Human enterocyte (CaCo-2) migration is modulated in vitro by extracellular matrix composition and epidermal growth factor. *Journal of Clinical Investigation* **90:** 15–23.

Beaulieu JF & Vachon PH (1994) Reciprocal expression of laminin A-chain isoforms along the crypt–villus axis in the human small intestine. *Gastroenterology* **106:** 829–839.

Burgeson RE, Chiquet M, Deutzmann R et al (1994) A new nomenclature for the laminins. *Matrix Biology* **14:** 209–211.

Burgess WH & Maciag T (1989) The heparin-binding (fibroblast) growth factor family of proteins. *Annual Review of Biochemistry* **58:** 575–606.

Carroll KM, Wong TT, Drabik DL & Chang EB (1988) Differentiation of rat small intestinal epithelial cells by extracellular matrix. *American Journal of Physiology* **254:** G355–G360.

Chinery R, Poulsom R, Rogers L et al (1992) Localization of intestinal trefoil-factor mRNA in rat stomach and intestine by hybridization in situ. *Biochemical Journal* **285:** 5–8.

Ciacci C, Lind SE & Podolsky DK (1993a) Transforming growth factor β regulation of migration in wounded rat intestinal epithelial monolayers. *Gastroenterology* **105:** 93–101.

Ciacci C, Mahida YR, Dignasss A et al (1993b) Functional interleukin-2 receptors on intestinal epithelial cells. *Journal of Clinical Investigation* **92:** 527–532.

Colgan SP, Resnick MB, Parkos CA et al (1994) IL-4 directly modulates function of a model human intestinal epithelium. *Journal of Immunology* **153:** 2122–2129.

Cook GA, Yeomans ND & Giraud AS (1995) Trefoil peptide expression falls following gastric mucosal injury but is induced in a TGFα-dependent manner late in repair. *Gastroenterology* **108:** A75 (abstract).

Dignass AU & Podolsky DK (1993) Cytokine modulation of intestinal epithelial cell restitution: central role of transforming growth factor β. *Gastroenterology* **105:** 1323–1332.

Dignass AU, Tsunekawa S & Podolsky DK (1994a) Fibroblast growth factors modulate intestinal epithelial cell growth and migration. *Gastroenterology* **106:** 1254–1262.

Dignass A, Lynch-Devaney K, Kindon H et al (1994b) Trefoil peptides promote epithelial migration through a transforming growth factor β-independent pathway. *Journal of Clinical Investigation* **94:** 376–383.

Dignass AU, Lynch-Devaney K & Podolsky DK (1994c) Hepatocyte growth factor/scatter factor modulates intestinal epithelial proliferation and migration. *Biochemical and Biophysical Research Communications* **202:** 701–709.

Eckmann L, Jung HC, Schürer-Maly C et al (1993) Differential cytokine expression by human intestinal epithelial cell lines: regulated expression of interleukin 8. *Gastroenterology* **105:** 1689–1697.

Ehrig K, Leivo I, Argraves WS et al (1990) Merosin, a tissue-specific basement membrane protein, is a laminin-like protein. *Proceedings of the National Academy of Sciences of the USA* **87:** 3264–3268.

Feil W, Wenzl E, Vattay P et al (1987) Repair of rabbit duodenal mucosa after acid injury in vivo and in vitro. *Gastroenterology* **92:** 1973–1986.

Feil W, Klimesch S, Karner P et al (1989a) Importance of an alkaline microenvironment for rapid restitution of the rabbit duodenal mucosa in vitro. *Gastroenterology* **97:** 112–122.

Feil W, Lacy ER, Wong YMM et al (1989b) Rapid epithelial restitution of human and rabbit colonic mucosa. *Gastroenterology* **97:** 685–701.

Gerecke DR, Wagman DW, Champliaud MF & Burgeson RE (1994) The complete primary structure for a novel laminin chain, the laminin B1 k chain. *Journal of Biological Chemistry* **269:** 11 073–11 080.

Göke M, Zuk A & Podolsky DK (1996) Regulation and function of extracellular matrix in intestinal epithelial restitution in vitro. *American Journal of Physiology* (in press).

Hahn U, Schuppan D, Hahn EG et al (1987) Intestinal cells produce basement membrane proteins in vitro. *Gut* **28:** S143-S151.

Hahn U, Stallmach A, Hahn EG & Riecken EO (1990) Basement membrane components are potent promoters of rat intestinal epithelial cell differentiation in vitro. *Gastroenterology* **98:** 322–335.

Hanby AM, Poulsom R, Singh S et al (1993) Spasmolytic polypeptide is a major antral peptide: distribution of the trefoil peptides human spasmolytic polypeptide and pS2 in the stomach. *Gastroenterology* **105:** 1110–1116.

Harvath L, Brownson NE, Fields GB & Skubitz APN (1994) Laminin peptides stimulate human neutrophil motility. *Journal of Immunology* **152:** 5447–5456.

Housley RM, Morris CF, Boyle W et al (1994) Keratinocyte growth factor induces proliferation of hepatocytes and epithelial cells throughout the rat gastrointestinal tract. *Journal of Clinical Investigation* **94:** 1764–1777.

Jeffrey GP, Oates PS, Wang TC et al (1994) Spasmolytic polypeptide: a trefoil peptide secreted by rat gastric mucous cells. *Gastroenterology* **106:** 336–345.

Jørgensen KH, Thim L & Jacobsen HE (1982) Pancreatic spasmolytic polypeptide (PSP): I. Preparation and initial chemical characterization of a new polypeptide from porcine pancreas. *Regulatory Peptides* **3:** 207–219.

Jung HC, Eckmann L, Yang SK et al (1995) A distinct array of proinflammatory cytokines is expressed in human colon epithelial cells in response to bacterial invasion. *Journal of Clinical Investigation* **95:** 55–65.

Kindon H, Pothoulakis C, Thim L et al (1995) Trefoil peptide protection of intestinal epithelial barrier function: cooperative interaction with mucin glycoprotein. *Gastroenterology* **109:** 516–523.

Koyama S & Podolsky DK (1989) Differential expression of transforming growth factors α and β in rat intestinal epithelial cells. *Journal of Clinical Investigation* **83:** 1768–1773.

Kurokawa M, Lynch K & Podolsky DK (1987) Effects of growth factors on an intestinal epithelial cell line: transforming growth factor β inhibits proliferation and stimulates differentiation. *Biochemical and Biophysical Research Communications* **142:** 775–782.

Lacy ER (1988) Epithelial restitution in the gastrointestinal tract. *Journal of Clinical Gastroenterology* **10 (supplement 1):** S72–S77.

Laurie GW, Leblond CP & Martin GR (1982) Localization of type IV collagen, laminin, heparan sulfate proteoglycan, and fibronectin to the basal lamina of basement membranes. *Journal of Cell Biology* **95:** 340–344.

Lipkin M, Sherlock P & Bell B (1963) Cell proliferation kinetics in the gastrointestinal tract of man. II. Cell renewal in stomach, ileum, colon, and rectum. *Gastroenterology* **45:** 721–729.

McCormack SA, Viar MJ & Johnson LR (1992) Migration of IEC-6 cells: a model for mucosal healing. *American Journal of Physiology* **263:** G426–G435.

Marinkowich MP, Lunstrom GP, Keene DR & Burgeson RE (1992) The dermal–epidermal junction of the human skin contains a novel laminin variant. *Journal of Cell Biology* **119:** 695–703.

Mashimo H, Podolsky DK & Fishman MC (1995) Structure and expression of murine intestinal trefoil factor: high evolutionary conservation and postnatal expression. *Biochemical and Biophysical Research Communications* **210:** 31–37.

Mayer L & Shlien R (1987) Evidence for function of Ia molecules on gut epithelial cells in man. *Journal of Experimental Medicine* **166:** 1471–1483.

Mayer L, Eisenhardt D, Salomon P et al (1991) Expression of class II molecules on intestinal epithelial cells in humans. Differences between normal and inflammatory bowel disease. *Gastroenterology* **100:** 3–12.

Moore R, Carlson S & Madara JL (1989) Rapid barrier restitution in an in vitro model of intestinal epithelial injury. *Laboratory Investigation* **60:** 237–244.

Moore R, Madri J, Carlson S & Madara JL (1992) Collagens facilitate epithelial migration in restitution of native guinea pig intestinal epithelium. *Gastroenterology* **102:** 119–130.

Moore R, Madara JL & MacLeod RJ (1994) Enterocytes adhere preferentially to collagen IV in a differentially regulated divalent cation-dependent manner. *American Journal of Physiology* **266:** G1099–G1107.

Nishida T, Nakagawa S, Awata T et al (1983) Fibronectin promotes epithelial migration of cultured rabbit cornea in situ. *Journal of Cell Biology* **97:** 1653–1657.

Nusrat A, Delp C & Madara JL (1992) Intestinal epithelial restitution. Characterization of a cell culture model and mapping of cytoskeletal elements in migrating cells. *Journal of Clinical Investigation* **89:** 1501–1511.

Nusrat A, Parkos CA, Bacarra AE et al (1994) Hepatocyte growth factor/scatter factor effects on epithelia. *Journal of Clinical Investigation* **93:** 2056–2065.

O'Keefe EJ, Payne RE, Russell N & Woodley DT (1985) Spreading and enhanced motility of human keratinocytes on fibronectin. *Journal of Investigative Dermatology* **85:** 125–130.

Olson AD, Pysher T & Bienkowski RS (1991) Organization of intestinal epithelial cells into multicellular structures requires laminin and functional actin microfilaments. *Experimental Cell Research* **192:** 543–549.

Paimela H, Goddard PJ, Carter K et al (1993) Restitution of frog gastric mucosa in vitro: effect of basic fibroblast growth factor. *Gastroenterology* **104:** 1337–1345.

Planchon SM, Martins CAP, Guerrant RL & Roche JK (1994) Regulation of intestinal epithelial barrier function by TGF-β1. *Journal of Immunology* **153:** 5730–5739.

Podolsky DK & Babyatsky MW (1995) Growth and development of the gastrointestinal tract. In Yamada T (ed.) *Textbook of Gastroenterology*, pp 546–577. Philadelphia: JB Lippincott.

Podolsky DK, Lynch-Devaney K, Stow JL et al (1993) Identification of human intestinal trefoil factor. Goblet-cell specific expression of a peptide targeted for apical secretion. *Journal of Biological Chemistry* **268:** 6694–6702.

Potten CS, Owen G, Hewitt D et al (1995) Stimulation and inhibition of proliferation in the small intestinal crypts of the mouse after in vivo administration of growth factors. *Gut* **36:** 864–873.

Quaroni A, Isselbacher KJ & Ruoshlahti (1978) Fibronectin synthesis by epithelial crypt cells of rat small intestine. *Proceedings of the National Academy of Sciences of the USA* **75:** 5548–5552.

Quaroni A, Wands J, Trelstad RL & Isselbacher KJ (1979) Epitheloid cell cultures from rat small intestine. Characterization by morphologic and immunologic criteria. *Journal of Cell Biology* **80:** 248–265.

Reinecker HC & Podolsky DK (1995) Human intestinal epithelial cells express functional cytokine receptors sharing the common γc chain of the interleukin 2 receptor. *Proceedings of the National Academy of Sciences of the USA* **92:** 8353–8357.

Rio MC, Bellocq JP, Daniel JY et al (1988) Breast-cancer associated pS2 protein: synthesis and secretion by normal stomach mucosa. *Science* **241:** 705–708.

Rio MC, Chenard MP, Wolf C et al (1991) Induction of pS2 and hSP genes as markers of mucosal ulceration of the digestive tract. *Gastroenterology* **100:** 375–379.

Ruoslahti E & Yamaguchi Y (1991) Proteoglycans as modulators of growth factor activities. *Cell* **64:** 867–869.

Rutten MJ & Ito S (1983) Morphology and electrophysiology of guinea pig gastric mucosal repair in vitro. *American Journal of Physiology* **244:** G171–G182.

Sarret Y, Stamm C, Jullien D & Schmitt D (1992) Keratinocyte migration is partially supported by the cell-binding domain of fibronectin and is RGDS-dependent. *Journal of Investigative Dermatology* **99:** 656–659.

Scott H, Solheim BG, Brandtzaeg P & Thorsby E (1980) HLA-DR-like antigens in the epithelium of the human small intestine. *Scandinavian Journal of Immunology* **12:** 77–82.

Selby WS, Janossy G, Mason DY & Jewell DP (1983) Expression of HLA-DR antigens by colonic epithelium in inflammatory bowel disease. *Clinical and Experimental Immunology* **53:** 614–618.

Silen W (1987) Gastric mucosal defense and repair. In Johnson LR (ed.) *Physiology of the Gastrointestinal Tract*, pp 1055–1069. New York: Raven Press.

Simo P, Simon-Assmann P, Arnold C & Kedinger M (1992a) Mesenchyme-mediated effect of dexamethasone on laminin in cocultures of embryonic gut epithelial cells and mesenchyme-derived cells. *Journal of Cell Science* **101:** 161–171.

Simo P, Bouziges F, Lissitzky JC et al (1992b) Dual and asynchronous deposition of laminin chains at the epithelial-mesenchymal interface in the gut. *Gastroenterology* **102:** 1835–1845.

Simon-Assmann P, Bouziges F, Freund JN et al (1990) Type IV collagen mRNA accumulates in the mesenchymal compartment at early stages of murine developing intestine. *Journal of Cell Biology* **110:** 849–857.

Simon-Assmann P, Duclos B, Orian-Rousseau V et al (1994) Differential expression of laminin isoforms and α6-β4 integrin subunits in the developing human and mouse intestine. *Developmental Dynamics* **201:** 71–85.

Steeb CB, Trahair JF & Read LC (1995) Administration of insulin-like growth factor-I (IGF-I) peptides for three days stimulates proliferation of the small intestinal epithelium in rats. *Gut* **37:** 630–638.

Stettler C, Schmassmann A, Poulsom R et al (1995) Effect of hepatocyte growth factor on expression of trefoil peptides in injured gastric mucosa. *Gastroenterology* **108:** A226 (abstract).

Suemori S, Ciacci C & Podolsky DK (1991a) Regulation of transforming growth factor expression in rat intestinal epithelial cell lines. *Journal of Clinical Investigation* **87:** 2216–2221.

Suemori S, Lynch-Devaney K & Podolsky DK (1991b) Identification and characterization of rat intestinal trefoil factor: tissue- and cell-specific member of the trefoil protein family. *Proceedings of the National Academy of Sciences of the USA* **88:** 11 017–11 021.

Taupin DR, Cook GA, Yeomans ND & Giraud AS (1994a) Increased trefoil peptide expression occurs late in the healing phase in a model of gastric ulceration in the rat. *Gastroenterology* **106:** A195 (abstract).

Taupin DR, Cook GA, Skultety KJ et al (1994b) Increased trefoil peptide expression in a rat model of intestinal repair. *Gastroenterology* **106:** A195 (abstract).

Thim L (1988) A surprising sequence homology. *Biochemical Journal* **253:** 309.

Thim L (1989) A new family of growth factor-like peptides. 'Trefoil' disulphide loop structures as a common feature in breast cancer associated peptide (pS2), pancreatic spasmolytic polypeptide (PSP), and frog skin peptides (spasmolysins). *FEBS Letters* **250**: 85–90.

Timpl R & Dziadek M (1986) Structure, development, and molecular pathology of basement membranes. *International Review of Experimental Pathology* **29**: 1–112.

Tomasetto C, Rio MC, Gautier C et al (1990) hSP, the domain-duplicated homolog of pS2 protein, is co-expressed with pS2 in stomach but not in breast. *EMBO Journal* **9**: 407–414.

Trier JS, Allan CH, Abrahamson DR & Hagen SJ (1990) Epithelial basement membrane of mouse jejunum. Evidence for laminin turnover along the entire crypt-villus axis. *Journal of Clinical Investigation* **86**: 87–95.

Turowski GA, Rashid Z, Hong F et al (1994) Glutamine modulates phenotype and stimulates proliferation in human colon cancer cells. *Cancer Research* **54**: 5974–5980.

Vachon PH & Beaulieu JF (1995) Extracellular heterotrimeric laminin promotes differentiation in human enterocytes. *American Journal of Physiology* **268**: G857–G867.

Vuolteenaho R, Nissinen M, Sainio K et al (1994) Human laminin M chain (merosin): complete primary structure, chromosomal assignment, and expression of the M and A chain in human fetal tissues. *Journal of Cell Biology* **124**: 381–394.

Waller DA, Thomas NW & Self TJ (1988) Epithelial restitution in the large intestine of the rat following insult with bile salts. *Virchows Archiv A. Pathological Anatomy and Histopathology* **414**: 77–81.

Weiser MM, Sykes DE & Killen PD (1990) Rat intestinal basement membrane synthesis. Epithelial versus nonepithelial contributions. *Laboratory Investigation* **62**: 325–330.

Wright NA, Poulsom R, Stamp GWH et al (1990) Epidermal growth factor (EGF/URO) induces expression of regulatory peptides in damaged human gastrointestinal tissues. *Journal of Pathology* **162**: 279–284.

Wright NA, Poulsom R, Stamp G et al (1993) Trefoil peptide gene expression in gastrointestinal epithelial cells in inflammatory bowel disease. *Gastroenterology* **104**: 12–20.

Yayon A, Klagsbrun M, Esko JD et al (1991) Cell surface, heparin-like molecules are required for binding of basic fibroblast growth factor to its high affinity receptor. *Cell* **64**: 841–848.

2

Antigen presentation in the intestine

ASIT PANJA
LLOYD MAYER

GENERAL ASPECTS OF ANTIGEN PRESENTATION

The immune system evolved as a mechanism for protecting the host from foreign pathogens. The hallmark of the immune system is its specificity and memory for substances it has encountered in the past. This specificity and memory are mediated by both cellular and soluble factors which come together to evoke a response. The cells regulating this process are both T and B lymphocytes. Both types of cell have receptors specific for a given antigen—a foreign protein, carbohydrate or lipid. They both possess the ability to expand (proliferate) when they encounter the specific antigen to which their receptors can bind. They also have the capacity to differentiate into effector cells: B cells secreting antibody, and T cells either killing (cytolytic) or secreting cytokines.

While both T and B cells recognize antigen through their respective receptors, the mechanism whereby this interaction occurs is distinct for the two types of cell. Surface immunoglobulin (antibody) on B cells will recognize antigens that are either free in solution or on surfaces. Antibody can bind to large macromolecules, intact bacteria and viruses without requiring the antigen to be altered in any fashion. In contrast, the receptor on T cells requires that the antigen be processed into a form that can be recognized by the receptor. Intact macromolecules, bacteria or viruses cannot be seen in their native state and, until recently, T cells were thought to be capable of recognizing only protein antigens. Furthermore, the T cell antigen receptor (TcR) is only capable of recognizing processed antigens when they are bound to one in a series of 'self' proteins which are genetically encoded in the major histocompatibility complex (MHC). Part of the TcR binds to the peptide and another part binds to components of the MHC (i.e. HLA A, B, C or D in man, H-2, I-A, I-E in mouse). This difference in the ability of T and B cells to recognize antigen leads to the requirement of an additional cell to interact with T cells. This group of cells has been termed antigen-presenting cells (APCs) for their ability to process larger macromolecules into smaller recognizable peptides and their ability to present these processed peptides in the context of an MHC molecule.

Baillière's Clinical Gastroenterology—
Vol. 10, No. 3, September 1996
ISBN 0–7020–2187–3
0950–3528/96/030407 + 19 $12.00/00

Two types of APC have been defined: (i) professional APCs, i.e. those that can take up antigen from the environment, process it through an endo-lysosomal pathway, and complex processed peptides to class II MHC molecules; and (ii) non-professional APCs, which do not constitutively express MHC class II but which can be induced to do so. Only B cells, monocytes/macrophages and dendritic cells are in the former category. There is a growing list of cells in the latter group. There are two pathways for antigen to enter a cell. Antigens can be engulfed by a phagocytic APC (macrophage) in a so-called exogenous pathway, or an organism can infect an APC and antigens can be generated within the cell (endogenous pathway).

In the exogenous pathway, larger macromolecules are internalized and broken down into smaller immunogenic peptides by acidic proteases within the endosomes of the APC. These 'processed' peptides (usually 10–14 amino acids in length) classically bind to MHC class II molecules and are expressed on the APC surface where they can contact the TcR on specific T cells.

The endogenous pathway is different in that antigens are generated within the cell as a result of viral or bacterial infection or malignant trans-formation. Intracellular pathogens utilize the host's cellular machinery to generate peptides used in the viral or bacterial life cycle. Peptides generated within the cytoplasm are processed by a series of proteolytic enzymes called proteosomes (e.g. LMP2, LMP7). Such peptides are then transported to the endoplasmic reticulum (by TAP proteins) where they can bind to newly formed MHC class I molecules. The peptide–MHC complex is then transported to the cell surface where it can be recognized by the TcR. Almost all nucleated cells express class I molecules and hence can present antigen through this pathway. Classically, antigens bound to class I molecules are recognized by CD8+ cytotoxic/suppressor T cells, and the class II bound peptides are recognized by CD4+ helper T cells. This is due to the fact that the natural ligand for class I is CD8 itself and for class II it is CD4. Thus, the general rule of thumb for systemic immune responses is that antigens taken up by phagocytic cells and processed within the endolysosomal pathway will bind to MHC class II molecules and stimulate CD4+ helper T cells. Intracellular infections which result in cytoplasmic processing and transport through the endoplasmic reticulum will result in binding to MHC class I molecules and activation of CD8+ suppressor/cyto-toxic cells.

There have been some recent findings which have brought this concept into question. While it was initially thought that all antigen presentation was accomplished by MHC class I or class II molecules, several non-classical MHC molecules (e.g. CD1, TL, Qa) have been described and have also been shown to have the capacity to present antigen. The types of cells which express non-classical MHC molecules are, in many cases, markedly different from professional APCs. For instance, CD1c is detected on thymocytes, dendritic cells, activated peripheral B cells and monocytes, while CD1d is expressed predominantly on the intestinal epithelium. In contrast to the classical MHC molecules (class I or class II),

CD1 molecules are non-polymorphic (Blumberg et al, 1991). Expression and presentation by mouse CD1 do not depend on TAP proteins (Holcombe et al, 1995). Furthermore, non-protein antigens have been shown to bind to, and to be presented by, non-classical MHC molecules. For example, Beckman et al (1994) demonstrated that human CD1b molecules can present non-peptide bacterial ligands such as mycolic acid (lipids). Using a peptide display library, Castano et al (1995) demonstrated that CD1 could bind peptides as well, although these were generally larger in length than those peptides bound by classical MHC molecules. The antigen-presenting function of other non-classical MHC molecules has been suggested by the observation that CTL can respond to TL antigens (Morita et al, 1994). However, the biological significance of this finding is not certain at this time. Hammer et al (1992, 1993) were unsuccessful in demonstrating any binding to peptide to TL antigens, using the same strategy for peptide binding as that successfully used with class I molecules.

The family of antigen-presenting cells

The role of the antigen-presenting cell in the process of an immune response is quite important. These cells provide the means for antigen recognition by immunocompetent T cells, and certain specialized APCs present antigen to B cells in the germinal centres in the lymph node (follicular dendritic cells). There are several clearly defined types of cell which have been shown to function as APCs. Common to all APCs is their ability to express (constitutively or induced) MHC class II molecules. Regardless of the fact that most of our knowledge is confined to in vitro phenomena, distinct differences exist among different APCs relating to their mechanism of antigen presentation. APCs act as accessory cells through a combination of antigen presentation (MHC/peptide), cytokine (IL1, IL6, TNF) production and the provision of secondary co-stimulatory signals for the amplification of T cell responses (e.g. B7/CD28, CD40/gp39). Macrophages are well-characterized APCs which are derived from circulating monocytes—part of the reticulo-endothelial system of phagocytic cells. Monocytes leave the blood stream and migrate to lymph nodes and spleen, where they develop into macrophages. These cells are large (16–20 μm), with active lysosomes, endosomes and hydrolytic enzymes. These phagocytes are not only essential for the initiation of immune reactions, but they also play a decisive role in T-cell activation through their ability to produce powerful accessory cytokines. In some organs, macrophages restrict their mobility and become permanent residents, such as the Kupffer cells in the liver or alveolar macrophages of the lung.

   B cells not only manifest their key role as antibody-producing cells, but also play a dual role in the immune response. They possess phagocytic capacity, through the interaction of specific antigen with sIg or complement (C3b and C3d) receptors, and can function as an APC. When an antigen comes into contact with sIg on the B cell, the antigen is internalized in an endocytic vacuole. It is then partially digested (processed) and presented, complexed to MHC class II determinants, to helper T cells. This activated T cell in turn produces essential cytokines needed for B cells to become antibody-producing plasma cells. Antigen-specific B cells may be the most efficient APCs. Terminally differentiated B cells lose their ability to serve as APCs.

Steinman and Cohn (1973) characterized another unique cell, the dendritic cell from mouse spleen, which has been demonstrated to be the most potent APC. Readily distinguishable from macrophages and B cells, the morphological features of dendritic cells are distinct in two respects. Dendritic cells lack lysosomes but do possess a set of endocytic vacuoles that may be specialized for antigen presentation rather than antigen scavenging. The other feature is that dendritic cells are actively motile, constantly forming and retracting long cell processes, veils, or dendrites. Dendritic cells express very high levels of MHC class II antigens but no Fc receptors (Steinman and Nussenzweig, 1980). These cells are powerful stimulators in a mixed lymphocyte response and, on a cell-per-cell basis, the most effective APCs characterized to date. These cells are present within lymph nodes, spleen, thymus, skin and the gastrointestinal tract. Depending upon the location, dendritic cells are part of a family of APCs that initiate local immune reactions. In the skin, these are the classical Langerhan cells; in the gut, they are represented by the veiled cells in Peyer's patch (see the following section). However, in contrast to macrophages and B cells, dendritic cells are not as efficient at uptake and processing of antigen.

Monocytes/macrophages, dendritic cells and B cells possess all the classical features of an APC, i.e. they express MHC class II molecules, are capable of endocytosis, and process and present antigen to T cells. These three types of cell have been termed 'professional APCs'.

Attention has recently been drawn to 'non-professional APCs' which activate T cell populations in a manner distinct from the interactions described above. Cells which have been so categorized are: activated human T cells, fibroblasts, endothelial cells, keratinocytes and a variety of other epithelial cells. These cells are capable of expressing MHC class II molecules (when activated), presenting peptides to T cells, or initiating allogeneic immune responses. However, the responses are distinct from those seen with professional APC–T cell interactions. For example, activated human T cells can express class II molecules (Lanzavecchia et al, 1988; Siliciano et al, 1988) and can take up, process, and present some proteins (human immunodeficiency virus (HIV) gp 120) to other T cells. However, activated T cells are incapable of presenting soluble antigen (e.g. tetanus toxoid) to T cells (Lanzavecchia et al, 1988) and the use of these cells as APCs usually results in the induction of anergy (LaSalle et al, 1992). Class II antigen expression has been induced on fibroblasts, endothelial cells, and a variety of epithelial cells including those of the intestine. Despite the fact that the class II molecules can be recognized by the T cell receptor, these cells either stimulate poorly or produce an unusual immune reaction. The neo-expression of class II molecules on epithelial cells in the thyroid or the pancreatic islets has been invoked to explain the induction of autoimmunity in these organs (Botazzo et al, 1993; Piccinini et al, 1987), with the presentation of self peptides to previously tolerized self-reactive T cells. This field of research is growing rapidly, and our understanding of the regulation of immune responses using such cells is expanding. One such cell, the intestinal epithelial cell, is described in greater depth in a subsequent section.

MECHANISMS OF ANTIGEN UPTAKE

Antigen presentation by APCs involves several steps. These include contact with the antigen, uptake or internalization, processing, and binding of processed peptide to the appropriate MHC molecule through which the T cell receptor can recognize it.

In the peripheral blood system antigen uptake can be achieved in two major ways: (1) receptor-(sIg, FcR, complement)-mediated, and (2) non-receptor-mediated phagocytosis or pinocytosis.

Receptor-mediated endocytosis

Receptor-mediated endocytosis is the most efficient and selective process of antigen uptake. The receptors which are involved in antigen uptake are either surface immunoglobulin receptors (sIg) on B cells and/or Fc receptors (FcR) and complement receptors (see below) on both B cells and monocytes/macrophages. sIg receptors bind only to specific antigens. Fc receptors also demonstrate selectivity with regard to Ig isotype and vary in their ability to bind with immune complexes. In both cases, when an antigen binds with these receptors, the receptor-bound antigen or immune complex is internalized in small vesicles called coated pits. Once internalized, several pathways are possible. The vesicle or early endosome acidifies, dissociates the complex, and the receptor either recycles to the surface or the endosome progresses further into the cytoplasm, fusing with vacuoles containing class II molecules. The late endosome (multivesicular body) is the site where proteases are activated, proteins are processed into small peptides and class II–peptide complexes are formed. Late endosomes fuse either with lysosomes or with the plasma membrane, allowing for surface expression of the class II–peptide complexes.

Chesnut and Grey (1981) showed the ability of rabbit IgG-specific B cells to present processed rabbit IgG to T cells. This way of producing a specific immune reaction is very effective. If antigen-specific B cells are presenting to antigen-specific T cells, help for clonal growth or differentiation (specific and non-specific) can be concentrated on these activated B cells. Rock and colleagues (1984) have reported that hapten-specific B lymphocytes are very efficient at presenting hapten to T cells after hapten binding to surface Ig molecules. In contrast to the requirements for non-specific antigen uptake by B cells, maximal stimulation of responding T lymphocytes can be achieved with a minimum of antigen (Chesnut et al, 1982) if the Ig receptor is utilized.

All professional APCs except dendritic cells, which are non-phagocytic, express Fc receptors. These receptors seem to play an important role in an immune response, making antigen uptake easier after binding to an immune complex. In this regard, Cohen and coworkers (1973) demonstrated that cytophilic antibodies in the serum of immune animals could improve the antigen-presenting capability of native macrophages. Celis and Chang (1984) reported similar results, and Kehry and Yamashita (1990) later supported this observation by showing that presentation of trinitrophenol (TNP) carrier conjugates by mouse B cells could be enhanced 100- to 1000-fold if TNP-specific IgE was bound to FcεRII on mouse B cells.

Antigen uptake by complement receptors

The complement system consists of about 25 plasma proteins which normally circulate in the blood in an inactive state. When a microorganism gains access to the body, complement components are activated in one of two orderly sequences (classical (Ig-mediated) and alternate complement cascade) which results in enhanced phagocytosis (opsonization) by B cells and macrophages. Complement is a major component of non-specific (innate) immunity, but it has been usurped by the adaptive immune system to enhance the effectiveness of specific immunity. The complement cascade can be activated through two pathways. The classical pathway evolved to be capable of interactions with components of the adaptive immune system as it depends upon the binding of antibodies to the invading organisms which subsequently binds to the C1 complex, initiating a series of enzymatic reactions (serine esterases). In the absence of an adaptive immune response (i.e. antibody), the alternative pathway is triggered by an interaction between bacterial components and C3 protein of the complement cascade, resulting in the generation of C3b fragments which coat bacteria. C3b receptors are expressed on macrophages and facilitate opsonization of these coated bacteria. The C3b receptor also can opsonize immune complexes (IgG and IgM) which have associated with C3b and, as such, prevents potential tissue injury from products of complement activation within the tissue. C3b receptors have also been shown to be present on red blood cells (Daha and van Es, 1984) which appear to facilitate complement-bound immune complex delivery to the Kupffer cells in the liver. In addition, it has been shown that the triggering of tetanus toxoid antigen-specific T cells by Epstein–Barr virus-transformed B cells can be enhanced by binding C3b and C4b components to the antigen. Thus, through a number of actions, complement can serve as a major mechanism involved in antigen uptake.

Phagocytosis and pinocytosis

Unlike receptor-(sIg, Fc or complement)-mediated endocytosis, which works in a very restricted fashion, phagocytosis and pinocytosis is a non-specific mechanism of antigen uptake. As noted earlier, monocytes/

macrophages, neutrophils and B cells are the common phagocytic cells in the human body. These cells protect the host by engulfing and disposing of bacteria and other foreign substances. When a foreign pathogen is encountered by a phagocyte, it is captured by cytoplasmic extensions (like an amoeba engulfs its food). It is then pulled inside the cytoplasm, and a membrane-lined vacuole (phagosome) is formed around it. This newly formed phagosome is then fused with a lysosome (phagolysosome). The antigen in the phagolysosome is partially degraded and peptide fragments are displayed on the APC surface coupled to MHC protein.

Similar to most other cells in the body, pinocytosis occurs in various cells in the intestinal tract. This is the manner by which nutrient absorption occurs. Both phagocytosis and pinocytosis are relatively inefficient and only a small proportion of antigen is taken up through this process. However, by either of these processes, antigen becomes incorporated into the endosomal compartment, where processing begins in an effort to generate a specific response.

THE MECHANISMS OF ANTIGEN PROCESSING

As alluded to earlier, there are at least two pathways involved in antigen processing. The first involves exogenous antigens which are endocytosed into acidic vesicles and degraded into peptides of appropriate length to allow for complexing with MHC class II, re-expression on the cell surface and recognition by the TcR (Margulies and Germain, 1993). Both class I and class II molecules are produced in the endoplasmic reticulum (ER). However, unlike MHC class I molecules, class II molecules do not bind peptides in this compartment. This is due to the fact that there is an additional protein which complexes with the class II molecule in the ER called invariant chain. Invariant chain essentially covers the antigen-binding cleft in the class II molecule and prevents any endogenously processed peptides from binding. Invariant chain is cleaved from the class II molecule in the acidic late endosome allowing for peptides resulting from exogenous uptake and processing to bind. Vacuoles containing class II molecules leave the ER and Golgi to fuse with late endosomes. Class I molecule-containing vacuoles leave the Golgi to fuse with the surface membrane. This clever mechanism essentially allows for the maintenance of the CD4–class II and CD8–class I dichotomy described earlier.

The other pathway involves endogenously synthesized antigens which are foreign proteins produced within a cell (such as viral proteins produced in infected cells or neo-antigens generated by malignant cells). These endogenous antigens are processed in the cytosol by proteosomes and transported by special proteins called TAPs (transporter associated with antigen processing) into the endoplasmic reticulum. There they bind to naked newly formed class I MHC molecules and migrate to the plasma membrane to present peptides to the TcR.

FACTORS CONTROLLING APC FUNCTION

As we have already discussed, the efficiency or specificity of antigen handling varies in different APCs. Although the mechanisms which regulate APC function are not yet fully understood, the role of cytokines on APC activity has been ascertained by a number of studies. In particular, γIFN has been shown to enhance phagocytosis and to upregulate the MHC class I or class II expression in both professional and non-professional APC (Rhodes et al, 1986), thus increasing the efficiency of antigen uptake and presentation. Another cytokine, GM-CSF, has been shown to enhance class II expression in monocytes (Willman et al, 1989; Chantry et al, 1990) and on a variety of epithelial cells. The expression of ICAM-1 and LFA-1 adhesion molecules has also been reported to be increased by γIFN and thus to enhance the adhesion between the T cell and the APC (Griffiths et al, 1989; Nikoloff and Griffiths, 1989; Renkonen, 1989). The influence of cytokines has also been demonstrated with regard to the co-stimulatory function of APCs. The expression of B7, which is expressed on conventional APCs and serves as ligand for CD28 on T cells can be enhanced by γIFN. On the other hand, some cytokines, such as TGFβ and IL-10, can have the opposite effects on the APC as both of these cytokines have been shown to down-regulate MHC class II expression on various APCs. Also, IL-10 has been shown to counter γIFN-induced B7 expression on monocytes resulting in anergy instead of an active immune response (Willems et al, 1994).

ANTIGEN-PRESENTING CELLS IN THE INTESTINE

The gastrointestinal (GI) tract is continually exposed to a variety of antigens in the lumen (resident bacteria, viruses, dietary). Defence mechanisms in the GI tract are therefore uniquely designed to deal with this constant insult. There are a number of non-immune non-specific physical and chemical barriers. Mucus-producing cells are present throughout the GI tract, and mucus has a protective role—preventing micro-organisms from attaching to the epithelium. Epithelial cells, which turn over every 24–96 hours in the small intestine, form tight junctions preventing access of antigen to the immunoreactive cells on the lamina propria. The chemical barriers which exist include gastric acid, bacteriostatic agents such as lysozyme, bacterocidal factors such as bile salts, proteases etc. These non-immune mechanisms are potent in their functional capacity to exclude antigens.

However, despite the fact that these non-specific barriers exist in the gut, the intestine is exposed to a tremendous antigenic load on a daily basis (dietary proteins and pathogens). In fact, a number of studies (Berg, 1992; Wells et al, 1993; van Leeuwen et al, 1994) have reported that non-pathogenic and pathogenic antigens (bacteria, parasites) can break the physical mucosal barrier. The intestinal immune system has the dilemma of trying to produce an active immune response to pathogens while, at the same time, preventing hypersensitivity to dietary antigens.

The intestinal immune system

The lamina propria of the stomach and intestine (including the colon) contains many lymphocytes and plasma cells. Some of these cells synthesize and secrete secretory IgA which has a role in protecting mucosal surfaces from bacterial invasion. Secretory IgA, the predominant immunoglobulin in the mucosa-associated lymphoid tissue, is produced locally by plasma cells as a dimeric molecule, and is taken up by mucosal epithelial cells via its interaction with secretory component. Secretory component serves not only as a transport pathway but also protects sIgA from digestive enzymes. Secretory IgA functions in part by preventing bacteria and viruses from binding to the epithelium.

Like any immune response, that in the intestinal tract results from the conglomerate of interactions between T cells, B cells, antigen-presenting cells and antigen itself. Antigen uptake from the lumen appears to occur by multiple routes and this may dictate the type of immune response generated. In contrast to the systemic immune system, the immune system of the gastrointestinal tract has some unique features. While all of the functional components of intestinal immune system are not yet fully understood, certain cell populations are recognized as important participants in the mucosal immune network.

Antigen-presenting cells in mucosal tissues

Antigen sampling from the gut lumen was initially shown to occur through specialized epithelium or M cells. These specialized cells derive from the crypts of Lieberkuhn within the follicle-associated epithelium (FAE) or overlying Peyer's patches. These FAE or M cells can transport soluble antigens (Gardiner et al, 1995), viruses, bacteria and macromolecules from the lumen to the intra-epithelial space (Owen, 1977; Wolf et al, 1981; Sicinski et al, 1990; Trier, 1991; Sanderson and Walker, 1993). While the transport of antigen across M cells to the lymphoid population in Peyer's patch is well documented, the antigen-processing capacity of these cells is not clear. Although they possess acid phosphatase-containing pre-lysosomal and lysosomal compartments (Owen et al, 1986) through which antigen processing can occur in conventional APC, utilization of this pathway generally needs class II to render it effective as a stimulus for T cells. The presence of class II molecules on M cells depends upon the species studied. Immunohistochemical studies by Bjerke and Brandtzaeg (1988) on human epithelium showed that there were very few M cells in the human intestinal epithelium which express class II molecules and lysosomes essential for antigen processing and presentation. More recently, it has been reported that M cells in the mouse express class II MHC (Allan et al, 1993). Despite this, there are no confirmatory data that these cells can process antigens. Thus, while the pinocytic function of M cells is clear, there are several questions about their ability to act as true APCs. Therefore it appears that alternative antigen-presenting cells must be considered in this antigen-loaded environment.

Macrophages are usually present in the villus core and subepithelial space in the crypt of the small bowel, under the dome (M cell) overlying Peyer's patches and in the patch itself (Golder and Doe, 1983; Berken et al, 1987; Harvey and Jones, 1991). In fact, phagocytosis of *Giardia muris* trophozoites by mucosal macrophages has been observed by Owen et al (1981), and it has been postulated that organisms transported through M cells to the basal lamina are taken up by macrophages. Lause and Bockman (1981) were able to demonstrate ferritin uptake by Peyer's patch macrophages. Macrophages are also found in the lamina propria. These are a heterogeneous population in terms of their morphology and staining profile with various mAbs (Mahida et al, 1989). These authors have shown that macrophages located in the superficial lamina propria (just below the epithelium) are large, round and are strongly positive for acid phosphatase (ACP) and non-specific esterase (NSE). The macrophages in the basal lamina are irregular in shape and are either negative or weakly positive for ACP and NSE. This morphological and phenotypic heterogeneity has been reflected in a number of functional studies, and the general feeling has been that gut macrophages are weak or inactive accessory cells, or that these cells can inhibit antibody responses (Spalding and Griffin, 1986; Steinman and Nussenzweig, 1980). Several substances have been found within such macrophages, including DNA from damaged cells (Sawicki et al, 1977). These findings provide evidence that such cells can sample, detoxify via the release of superoxides and other chemical mediators and scavenge potentially harmful substances. Further evidence was provided by Joel et al (1978) who reported that when mice were fed carbon particles, a large amount of these particles accumulated in the subepithelial macrophages but not in the Peyer's patch.

As discussed above, dendritic cells are thought to be the most potent APC. Two groups of dendritic cells have been characterized in the gut. Sminia and Jeurissen (1986), Marsetyawan et al (1990) and Bland and Kambarage (1991) have reported classical dendritic cells which are esterase-negative, acid phosphatase-negative, FcR-negative, fibronectin non-adherent, and strongly DR-positive, with dendritic extensions that are actively engaged in T cell interactions. These cells are capable of stimulating mixed lymphocyte reactions (MLR; Mahida et al, 1988). The second group of dendritic cells are interdigitating cells (also known as veiled cells) located in Peyer's patches which stain with 33D1, an anti-dendritic cell monoclonal antibody (Nussenzweig et al, 1982; Meyerhofer et al, 1983). These cells are effective APCs. While the use of immunohistochemistry to define the tissue macrophage and dendritic cell populations in the gut has been of considerable value, difficulties in the isolation of dendritic cells has resulted in a poor estimation of the number of dendritic cells present or their functional role in the intestinal mucosa. Studies by Selby et al (1983) and Hume et al (1987) indicated that, in small bowel lamina propria, most of the DR⁺ histocytes are dendritic cells as they were weakly non-specific esterase-positive, and strongly membrane ATPase-positive. Work by Selby et al also suggested that small bowel DR⁺ cells act as antigen-presenting cells, whereas colonic accessory cells are more phagocytic.

Although the abundance of plasma cells in the lamina propria has been known for many years, the antigen-presenting role of B cells in this particular system has not been characterized. Recent studies by Brandtzaeg and colleagues hypothesized that specialized B cells in the M cell pocket facilitate antigen presentation and diversification of the mucosal immune response (Farstad et al, 1994).

So how does antigen-uptake occur, and which cells are responsible for antigen presentation in the gut? One candidate is the epithelial cell. For many years it has been known that food antigens cross the epithelium and can be detected in the serum (reviewed by Husby, 1988), supporting the capacity of intestinal epithelial cells (IEC) to take up antigen. Interestingly, a large number of studies reported that IECs could express (constitutively or induced) MHC class II molecules (Willman et al, 1978; Mason et al, 1981; Bland and Warren, 1986; Mayer and Shlien, 1987; Mowat, 1987; Kaiserlian et al, 1990; Salomon et al, 1991). More recently, several laboratories have shown that IECs are capable of processing and presenting antigens to immunocompetent T cells in vitro (Mayer and Shlien, 1987; Bland and Whiting, 1989; Hoyne et al, 1993). These findings fulfil the minimum requirements for IEC to be considered as potential APCs.

MHC class II expression by IEC

There is general agreement among investigators that IECs in the small intestine constitutively express class II molecules; however, controversy exists regarding the ability of colonocytes to express class II MHC. The constitutive expression in the small bowel may relate to the presence of activated IELs or LPLs (Cerf-Bensussan et al, 1984) and is increased in the conditions where γIFN is produced or passively administered (Quyang et al, 1988; Steiniger et al, 1989; Masson and Perdue, 1990; Zhang and Michael, 1990). Interestingly, the class II expressed by the IECs is present on both the luminal and basolateral surface, raising a question about its role in antigen presentation to T cells. Bland (1990) suggested that these class II molecules may serve as 'peptide receptors' for pre-digested or pre-processed peptides that result from luminal factors within the stomach and upper gastrointestinal tract. Studies by his group have also demonstrated that antigen uptake and processing by rat entero-cytes is slower and less efficient than in monocytes. Similar findings have been described by So et al (submitted) for human IEC and were further supported by studies in a rotavirus-infected animal model (Majerowicz et al, 1994) system. This group documented the presence of rotavirus particles in the viroplasm near the rough endoplasmic reticulum in enterocytes. Class II expression and antigen presentation by IEC may depend upon several other environmental factors. Recent studies by Sanderson and Walker, 1993) showed that expression of class II mRNA in mouse intestinal epithelium appeared to depend upon the introduction of a complex diet (foreign antigens).

Antigen uptake by IEC

The generation of an immune response by mucosal T cells would require antigen uptake by the epithelium. In the newborn, growth factors from milk are thought to be taken up by this process. IECs have also been studied in vitro for their ability to take up antigen. There is evidence that macromolecules can be taken up by the enterocytes through endocytosis (by binding to apical membrane) or pinocytosis (for soluble molecules). Gonella and Neutra (1984) have shown that both soluble and lectin-bound ferritin enters the vesicular system of neonatal ileal epithelial cells. However, only the lectin-bound molecules reached the basolateral membrane while nonbound molecules were destroyed in the lysosomal compartment. The binding of macromolecules seems to depend on the maturity of the enterocytes. A number of studies have shown that macromolecules, including bovine serum albumin (BSA) and horseradish peroxidase (HRP), are transported across IEC more readily in young animals and that this property decreases with age (Udall et al, 1981; Robertson et al, 1982; Teichberg et al, 1992). Lamm and colleagues (Kaetzel et al, 1991) showed in an in vitro model system that polymeric IgA, complexed to its specific antigen, can be transcytosed from the basolateral side of the epithelial cells via the polymeric Ig receptor to the epithelial cell surface. They proposed that this could be a mechanism for the clearance of antigens (which move through the epithelium) from the lamina propria to the lumen, or as a mechanism for the intracellular destruction of pathogens.

Once macromolecules are internalized in the membrane-bound compartments, the lysosomal enzymes (cathepsin B and D, acid phosphatase, mannosidase) break down antigens into smaller peptides. While these lysosome-derived intracellular enzymes are detectable throughout the intestine, there has been controversy as to whether epithelial cells actually have these molecules. Consistent with this are the findings of several studies which have documented the poor processing capacity of IECs. Some membrane-bound macromolecules may escape digestion in the lumen as well as within the cell and reach the basolateral surface intact.

Antigen entry through the epithelium can also occur by the paracellular route. In the healthy intestine, paracellular antigen uptake is limited as the pore size of the tight junctions between the epithelial cells is quite small (about 5 nm) and does not allow immunogenic polypeptides to pass through. However, in pathological settings epithelial integrity may become disrupted, and an increased pore size may allow for the passage of antigens. Indeed, Walker and colleagues (Bloch et al, 1979) showed that the serum level of BSA in fed animals is increased in the *Nippostrongylus*-infected rat when compared with controls. Similarly, Perdue and colleagues (Ramage et al, 1988) demonstrated an increase in the permeability to ^{51}Cr-labelled EDTA and ovalbumin in the acutely inflamed intestine. High levels of serum ovalbumin (after oral challenge) are observed in infants recovering from gastroenteritis. Once antigen travels between the epithelium, sub-epithelial macrophages can take up, process and present antigen to lamina propria T cells.

CD8$^+$ T cell stimulation by IEC

Several unique features of IECS set them apart from classical APCs. These include the selective activation of CD8$^+$ suppressor T cells (Bland and Warren, 1986; Mayer and Shlien, 1987) or suppression of immune response through soluble factors (PGE$_2$) (Santos et al, 1990). IECs are capable of stimulating CD4$^+$ T cells as well (Kaiserlian et al, 1990) although, in humans and rats, CD8$^+$ T cell proliferation predominates. Despite these in vitro findings there is no firm evidence that these cells act as APCs in vivo. It is clear that they participate in inflammatory processes (see below) and that they serve as conduits for products of the immune system (IgA). Directed in vivo studies will be required to address their true role in immunoregulation.

The potential role of non-classical MHC molecules in antigen presentation by IEC

While class I and II MHC molecules are the major regulators of antigen presentation, it has been thought that a group of non-classical class-I molecules is involved in the specific recognition of self and microbial antigens by a subset of T cells. Porcelli et al (1992) have reported that MHC-related CD1 proteins are capable of presenting antigen to immuno-competent T cells. These investigators generated a cell line of double negative (CD4/CD8-negative) peripheral blood T cells by stimulation with crude lysates of *Mycobacterium tuberculosis* and CD1-positive monocytes. Clones from these cell lines were responsive to *M. tuberculosis* only in the presence of CD1$^+$ monocytes from any donor. The proliferation of T cells in this system was blocked by anti-CD1b mAbs, but not by mAbs to other CD1 subtypes, MHC class I or class II proteins. Furthermore, the T cell response was inhibited by a prior formaldehyde fixation of the APC, indicating the need for a processed antigen in this system.

Thus, it is possible that non-classical MHC molecules may have important roles in the intestinal micro-environment. These molecules may also play a role in the activation of unique sets of T cells (IEL and LPL—see above).

Cytokine profile of IEC

One of the general properties of an APC is its ability to produce accessory cytokines. These cytokines are defined as regulatory in that they can either enhance (IL1, IL6, TNF) or inhibit (IL10, TGFβ) T cell activation or are pro-inflammatory (e.g. IL8, Gro α, MCP-1, MIP 1α). This property also applies to IECs. Several laboratories have shown that intestinal epithelial cells are capable of producing many of the cytokines (IL6, GMCSF) that are known to be associated with APC function in conventional APCs. However, the cytokine profile of IECs differs from that of conventional APCs in that they fail to produce IL-1β (Quyang et al, 1988; Panja et al, 1995a), a cytokine which is thought to be important for T cell activation. Some cytokines may exert inhibitory effects on the immune system, such as those ascribed to TGFβ. Koyama and Podolsky (1989) have reported the synthesis of TGFβ by IECs (cell lines), and the synthesis is triggered by 'wounding' or cell monolayers (Ciacci et al, 1993). We have reported the existence of IL-10 production by IECs in culture (Panja et al, 1995b). Both TGFβ and IL-10 have inhibitory effects on immune activation. Kagnoff and colleagues have documented that IEC lines (T84, CaCO2) are capable of synthesizing pro-inflammatory cytokines, such as IL8, especially in the presence of bacterial invasion (Eckmann et al, 1993a). IL8 mRNA expression and protein synthesis in culture has also been demonstrated in freshly isolated IECs by this group (Eckmann et al, 1993b). Lastly, GM-CSF, a cytokine which promotes antigen presentation by stimulating phagocytosis and class II antigen expression in macrophages (Panja et al, 1994), has been recently shown to be produced by IECs as well. Thus, IEC-derived cytokines may be involved in the regulation of multiple biological events via either autocrine or paracrine pathways on different target cells in the surrounding tissue. These cytokines may form a cascade or cytokine network regulating the APC function of IEC as well as other cells in the intestine.

Co-stimulatory molecule expression by IEC

Several molecules have been characterized as potent co-stimulatory molecules in conventional antigen-presenting cells. These include B7.1 (CD80) (a ligand for CD28 on T cells), B7.2 (CD86) (a ligand for CTLA4), intercelluiar adhesion molecule-1 (ICAM-1: the receptor for lymphocyte function associated molecule LFA-1) or cytokines (IL1, IL6, secreted or cell-bound). In the absence of secondary signals, resting T cells develop unresponsiveness (anergy) or tolerance to antigenic stimulation. Thus, APC provide a second signaling pathway which results in an active response to antigen. Epithelial cells generally fail to express many of these co-stimulatory molecules. Neither B7 nor ICAM-1 expression have been demonstrated in normal or inflamed IEC. Thus there is ample evidence that IECs can act as effective APCs, but yet lack a complete set of co-stimulatory signals (although it is not known whether physiologically related T cells, i.e. IEL or LPL, would require such secondary signals). A clear-cut documentation of antigen-presenting function by epithelial cell, as well as the mechanisms involved in vivo, is yet to be established.

SUMMARY

The intestinal mucosa is the largest surface area in the body which is continually exposed to an enormous amount of food antigens, viruses, bacteria, parasites or the by-products of these organisms. In such an antigen-loaded environment, specialized defence mechanisms must exist. There is clear evidence that the function of lymphocytes in the intestinal mucosa (IELs or LPLs) is different from that of lymphocytes of the peripheral blood, lymph node or spleen (these are antigen-free organs). The basic processes of these reactions are not completely understood. The role of differential antigen handling and presentation, and the non-random distribution of responsibilities between the professional and non-professional APC in this regard, have not been characterized. Thus, much remains to be learned about the basic mechanisms of antigen uptake, processing and presentation in the intestine which are necessary to induce an immune response. Diversity in APC function is a natural requirement for the maintenance of homeostasis in the intestine. Subpopulations of professional and non-professional APC may have been programmed to function in such a way that non-professional APCs may play a dominant role. It is anticipated that in vivo model systems will be developed and that eventually a clearer understanding will be gained in this rapidly evolving field.

Acknowledgements

Dr Panja is recipient of a career development award from the Crohn's and Colitis Foundation of America. This work was supported by US Public Health Service grants AI-23504, AI-24671 and DK-44156 (L. Mayer).

REFERENCES

Allan CH, Mendrick DL & Trier JS (1993) Rat intestinal M cells contain acidic endosomal–lysosomal compartments and express class II major histocompatibility complex determinants. *Gastroenterology* **104**: 697–708.

Beckman EM, Porcelli SA, Morita CT et al (1994) Recognition of a lipid antigen by CD1 restricted ab+ T cells. *Nature* **372**: 691.

Berg RD (1992) Bacterial translocation from the gastrointestinal tract. *Journal of Medicine* **23**: 217–244.

Berken W, Northwood I, Beliveau C & Gump D (1987) Phagocytes in cell suspensions of human colon mucosa. *Gut* **28**: 976–980.

Bjerke K & Brandtzaeg P (1988) Lack of relation between HLA-DR and secretory component (SC) in follicle associated epithelium of human Peyers patches. *Clinical and Experimental Immunology* **71**: 502–507.

Bland PW & Kambarage DM (1991) Antigen handling by the epithelium and lamina propria macrophages. *Gastroenterology Clinics of North America* **20**: 577.

Bland PW & Warren LG (1986) Antigen presentation by epithelial cells of the rat small intestine. I. Kinetics, antigen specificity and blocking by anti-Ia antisera. *Immunology* **58**: 1–7.

Bland PW & Whiting CV (1989) Antigen processing by isolated rat intestinal villus enterocytes. *Immunology* **68**: 497–502.

Bloch KJ, Bloch DB, Stern M & Walker WA (1979) Intestinal uptake of macromolecules. VI. Uptake of protein antigen in vivo in normal rats and rats infected with *Nippostrongylus brasiliensis* or subjected to mild systemic anaphylaxis. *Gastroenterology* **77**: 1038–1044.

Blumberg RS, Terhorst C, Bleicher P et al (1991) Expression of a non-polymorphic MHC class-I like molecule, CD1d, by human intestinal epithelial cells. *Journal of Immunology* **147**: 2518.

Botazzo GF, Pujol-Burrell R, Haanafusa T & Fleddman M (1993) Role of aberrant HLA-DR expression and antigen presentation in induction of endocrine autoimmunity. *Lancet* **ii**: 1115–1118.

Castano AR, Tangri S, Miller JE et al (1995) Mouse CD1 is an antigen presenting molecule with novel peptide binding properties. *Science* **269**: 223–226.

Celis E & Chang TW (1984) Antibodies to hepatitis B surface antigen potentiate the response of human T lymphocyte clones to the same antigen. *Science* **224**: 297–299.

Cerf-Bensussan N, Quaroni A, Kurnick J & Bhan A (1984) Intraepithelial lymphocytes modulate Ia expression by intestinal epithelial cells. *Journal of Immunology* **132**: 2244–2251.

Chantry D, Turner M, Brennan F et al (1990) Granulocyte–macrophage colony stimulating factor induces both HLA-DR expression and cytokine production by human monocytes. *Cytokine* **2**: 60–67.

Chesnut RW & Grey HM (1981) Studies on the capacity of B cells to serve as antigen presenting cells. *Journal of Immunology* **126**: 1075–1079.

Chesnut RW, Colon SM & Grey HM (1982) Antigen presentation by normal B cells, B cell tumors, and macrophages: functional and biochemical comparison. *Journal of Immunology* **128**: 1764–1768.

Ciacci C, Lind ES & Podolsky DK (1993) Transforming growth factor beta regulation of neutrophil migration in wounded rat intestinal epithelial monolayers. *Gastroenterology* **105**: 93–101.

Cohen BE, Rosenthal AK & Paul WE (1973) Antigen–macrophage interaction. II. Relative roles of cytophilic antibody and other membrane sites. *Journal of Immunology* **111**: 820–828.

Daha MR & van Es LA (1984) Fc- and complement receptor-dependent degradation of soluble immune complexes and stable immunoglobulin aggregates by guinea pig monocytes, peritoneal macrophages, and Kupffer cells. *Journal of Leukocyte Biology* **36**: 569–579.

Eckmann L, Jung HC, Schurer-Maly C et al (1993a) Differential cytokine expression by human intestinal epithelial cells: regulated expression of interleukin-8. *Gastroenterology* **105**: 1689–1697.

Eckmann L, Kagnoff MF & Fierer J (1993b) Epithelial cells secrete the chemokine interleukin-8 in response to bacterial entry. *Infection and Immunity* **61**: 4569–4574.

Farstad IN, Halstenson TS, Fausa I & Brandtzaeg P (1994) Heterogeneity of M cell associated B and T cells in human Peyer's patches. *Immunology* **83**: 457–464.

Fiocchi C (1989) Lymphokine and intestinal immune response. Role in inflammatory bowel disease. *Immunological Investigation* **18**: 91–102.

Gardiner KR, Anderson NH, Rowlands BJ & Darbul A (1995) Colitis and colonic mucosal barrier dysfunction. *Gut* **37**: 530–535.

Golder JP & Doe WF (1983) Isolation and preliminary characterization of human intestinal macrophages. *Gastroenterology* **84**: 795–802.

Gonnela PA & Neutra MR (1984) Membrane bound and fluid-phase macromolecules enter separate prelysosomal compartments in absorptive cells of suckling rat ileum. *Journal of Cell Biology* **99**: 909–917.

Griffiths CE, Voorhees JJ & Nickoloff BJ (1989) Characterization of intercellular adhesion molecule-1 and HLA-DR expression in normal and inflamed skin: modulation by recombinant gamma interferon and tumor necrosis factor. *Journal of the American Academy of Dermatology* **20**: 617–629.

Hammer J, Takacs B & Sinigaglia F (1992) Identification of a motif for HLA-DR1 binding peptides using M13 display libraries. *Journal of Experimental Medicine* **176**: 1007.

Hammer J, Valsasnini P, Tolba K et al (1993) Promiscuous and allele-specific anchors in HLA-DR binding peptides. *Cell* **74**: 197.

Harvey J & Jones DB (1991) Human mucosal T-lymphocyte and macrophage subpopulations in normal and inflamed intestine. *Clinical and Experimental Allergy* **21**: 549–560.

Holcombe HR, Castano AR, Chroutte H et al (1995) Non-classical behavior of the thymus leukemia antigen: peptide transporter-independent expression of a non-classical class-I molecule. *Journal of Experimental Medicine* **181**: 1433.

Hoyne GF, Callow MG, Kuo MC & Thomas WR (1993) Presentation of peptides and proteins by intestinal epithelial cells. *Immunology* **80**: 204–208.

Hume DA, Allan W, Hogan PG & Doe WF (1987) Immunohistochemical characterization of macrophages in human liver and gastrointestinal tract: expression of CD4, HLA-DR, OKM1, and the mature macrophage marker 25F9 in normal and diseased tissue. *Journal of Leukocyte Biology* **42**: 474–484.

Husby S (1988) Dietary antigens: uptake and humoral immunity in man. *Acta Pathologica Microbiologica et Immunologica Scandinavica* **1 (supplement)**: 1–40.

Joel DD, Laissue JA & LeFevre ME (1978) Distribution and fate of ingested carbon particles in mice. *Journal of Reticuloendothelial Society* **24**: 477.

Kaetzel CS, Robinson JK, Chintalacharuvu KR et al (1991) The polymeric immunoglobulin receptor (secretory component) mediates transport of immune complexes across epithelial cells: a local defense function for IgA. *Proceedings of the National Academy of Sciences of the USA* **88:** 8796–8800.

Kaiserlian D, Nicolas JF & Revillard JP (1990) Constitutive expression of Ia molecules by murine epithelial cells: a comparison between keratinocytes and enterocytes. *Journal of Investigative Dermatology* **94:** 385–386.

Kehry MR & Yamashita LC (1990) Role of the low affinity Fc epsilon receptor in B-lymphocyte antigen presentation. *Immunology* **141:** 77–81.

Koyama S & Podolsky DK (1989) Differential expression of transforming growth factors a and b in rat intestinal epithelial cells. *Journal of Clinical Investigation* **83:** 1768–1773.

Lanzavecchia A, Roosnek E, Gregory T et al (1988) T cells can present antigens such as HIV gp120 targeted to their own surface molecules. *Nature* **334:** 530–532.

LaSalle JM, Tolentino PJ, Freeman GJ et al (1992) Early signalling defects in human T cells anergized by T cell presentation of autoantigen. *Journal of Experimental Medicine* **176:** 177–186.

Lause DB & Bockman DE (1981) Heterogeneity, position, and functional capability of the macrophages in Peyer's patches. *Cell and Tissue Research* **218:** 557–566.

Mahida YR, Wu KC & Jewell DP (1988) Characterization of antigen-presenting activity of intestinal mononuclear cells isolated from normal and inflammatory bowel disease colon and ileum. *Immunology* **65:** 543–549.

Mahida YR, Patel S, Gionchetti P et al (1989) Macrophage subpopulations in lamina propria of normal and inflamed colon and terminal ileum. *Gut* **30:** 826–834.

Majerowicz S, Kubelka CF, Stephens P & Barth OM (1989) Ultrastructural study on experimental infection of rotavirus in a murine heterologous model. *Memorias Do Instituto Oswaldo Cruz* **89:** 395–402.

Margulies D & Germain R (1993) The biochemistry and cell biology of antigen presentation. *Annual Review of Immunology* **11:** 403–450.

Marsetyawan S, Biewenga J, Kraal G & Sminia T (1990) The localization of macrophage subsets and dendritic cells in the gastrointestinal tract of the mouse with special reference to the presence of high endothelial venules. *Cell and Tissue Research* **259:** 587–593.

Mason DW, Dallman M & Barclay AN (1981) Graft versus host disease induces expression of Ia antigen in rat epidermal cells and gut epithelium. *Nature* **293:** 150–151.

Masson SD & Perdue MH (1990) Changes in distribution of Ia antigen on epithelium of the jejunum and ileum in rats infected with *Nippostrongylus brasilienses*. *Clinical Immunology and Immunopathology* **57:** 83–95.

Mayer L & Shlien R (1987) Evidence for function of Ia molecules on gut epithelial cells in man. *Journal of Experimental Medicine* **166:** 1471–1483.

Meyerhofer G, Pugh CW & Barclay AN (1983) The distribution ontogeny and origin in the rat of Ia-positive cells with dendritic morphology and of Ia antigen in epithelia, with special reference to the intestine. *European Journal of Immunology* **13:** 112–122.

Morita A, Takahashi T, Stockert E et al (1994) TL antigen as a transplantation antigen recognized by TL-restricted cytotoxic T cells. *Journal of Experimental Medicine* **179:** 777.

Mowat AM (1987) The regulation of immune responses to dietary protein antigens. *Immunology Today* **8:** 93–98.

Nikoloff BJ & Griffiths CE (1989) T lymphocytes and monocytes bind to keratinocytes in frozen sections of biopsy specimens of normal skin treated with gamma interferon. *Journal of the American Academy of Dermatology* **20:** 736–743.

Nussenzweig MC, Steinman RM, Witmer MD & Gutchinov B (1982) A monoclonal antibody specific for mouse dendritic cells. *Proceedings of the National Academy of Sciences of the USA* **79:** 161–165.

Owen RL (1977) Sequential uptake of horseradish peroxidase by lymphoid follicle epithelium of Peyer's patches in the normal unobstructed mouse intestine: an ultrastructural study. *Gastroenterology* **72:** 440–451.

Owen RL, Allen CL & Stevens DP (1981) Phagocytosis of *Giardia muris* by macrophages in Peyer's patch epithelium in mice. *Infection and Immunity* **33:** 591–601.

Owen RL, Pierce NF, Apple RT & Cray WC Jr (1986) M cell transport of *Vibrio cholerae* from the intestinal lumen into Peyer's patch: a mechanism for antigen sampling and for microbial trans-epithelial migration. *Journal of Infectious Diseases* **153:** 1108–1118.

Panja A, Eckman L, Kagnoff MF & Mayer L (1994) Increased production of IL-8 and GM-CSF by intestinal epithelial cells in inflammatory bowel disease. *Gastroenterology* **106:** A750 (abstract).

Panja A, Siden E & Mayer L (1995a) Synthesis and regulation of accessory/proinflammatory cytokines by intestinal epithelial cells. *Journal of Clinical and Experimental Immunology* **100:** 298–305.

Panja A, Zhou Z, Mullin G & Mayer L (1995b) Secretion and regulation of IL-10 by intestinal epithelial cells. *Gastroenterology* **108:** A890 (abstract).

Piccinini LA, Goldsmith NK, Roman SH & Davies TF (1987) HLA-DP, DQ and DR gene expression in Graves disease and normal thyroid epithelium. *Tissue Antigens* **30:** 145–154.

Porcelli S, Morita CT & Brenner MB (1992) Cd1b restricts the response of human CD4-8-lymphocytes to a microbial antigen. *Nature* **360:** 593–597.

Quyang Q, El-Youssef M, Yen-Lieberman B et al (1988) Expression of HLA-DR antigens in inflammatory bowel disease mucosa: role of intestinal lamina propria mononuclear cell derived interferon gamma. *Digestive Disease and Sciences* **33:** 1528–1536.

Ramage JK, Stanisz A, Scicchitano R et al (1988) Effect of immunologic reactions on rat intestinal epithelium. Correlation of increased permeability to chromium 51-labeled ethylenediaminetetraacetic acid and ovalbumin during acute inflammation and anaphylaxis. *Gastroenterology* **94:** 1368–1375.

Renkonen R (1989) Regulation of intercellular adhesion molecule-1 expression on endothelial cells with correlation to lymphocyte-endothelial binding. *Scandinavian Journal of Immunology* **29:** 717–721.

Rhodes J, Ivanyi J & Cozens P (1986) Antigen presentation by human monocytes: effects of modifying major histocompatibility complex class II antigen expression and interleukin 1 production by using recombinant interferons and corticosteroids. *European Journal of Immunology* **16:** 370–375.

Robertson DM, Paganelli R, Dinwiddie R & Levinsky RJ (1982) Milk antigen absorption in the preterm and term neonate. *Archives of Disease in Childhood* **57:** 369–372.

Rock KL, Benacerraf B & Abbas AK (1984) Antigen presentation by hapten-specific B lymphocytes. I. Role of surface immunoglobulin receptors. *Journal of Experimental Medicine* **160:** 1102–1113.

Salomon P, Pizzimenti A, Panja A et al (1991) The expression and regulation of HLA-DR and HLA-DP in normal and inflammatory bowel disease peripheral blood monocytes and intestinal epithelial cells. *Autoimmunity* **9:** 141–149.

Sanderson IR & Walker WA (1993) Uptake and transport of macromolecules by the intestine: possible role in clinical disorders (an update). *Gastroenterology* **104:** 622–639.

Santos LM, Lider O, Audette J et al (1990) Characterization of immunomodulatory properties and accessory cell function of small intestinal epithelial cells. *Cellular Immunology* **127:** 26–34.

Sawicki W, Kucherczyk K, Szymanska K & Kujawa M (1977) Lamina propria macrophages of intestine of the guinea pig. *Gastroenterology* **73:** 1340–1344.

Selby WS, Poulter LW, Hobbs S et al (1983) Heterogeneity of HLA DR-positive histiocytes in human intestinal lamina propria: a combined histochemical and immunohistological analysis. *Journal of Clinical Pathology* **36:** 379–384.

Sicinski P, Rowinsky J, Warchol JB et al (1990) Poliovirus type 1 enters the human host through intestinal M cells. *Gastroenterology* **98:** 56–58.

Siliciano RF, Lawton T, Knall C et al (1988) Analysis of host virus interactions in AIDS with anti-gp120 T cell clones: effect of HIV sequence viration and a mechanism for CD4+ cell depletion. *Cell* **54:** 561–575.

Sminia T & Jeurissen SH (1986) The macrophage population of the gastrointestinal tract of the rat. *Immunobiology* **172:** 72–80.

Spalding DM & Griffin JA (1986) Different pathways of differentiation of pre-B cell lines are induced by dendritic cells and T cells from different lymphoid tissues. *Cell* **44:** 507.

Spalding DM, Williamson SI, Koopman WJ & McGhee JR (1984) Preferential induction of polyclonal IgA secretion by murine Peyer's patch dendritic T cell mixtures. *Journal of Experimental Medicine* **160:** 941–946.

Steiniger B, Falk P, Lohmuller M & van der Meide PH (1989) Class II MHC antigens in the rat digestive system. Normal distribution and induced expression after interferon gamma treatment in vivo. *Immunology* **68:** 507–513.

Steinman RM & Cohn Z (1973) Identification of a novel cell type in peripheral lymphoid organs of mice. I. Morphology, quantitation, tissue distribution. *Journal of Experimental Medicine* **137:** 1142–1162.

Steinman RM & Nussenzweig MC (1980) Dendritic cells: features and functions. *Immunological Review* **53:** 127–147.

Teichberg S, Wapnir RA, Moyse J & Lifshitz F (1992) Development of the neonatal rat small intestinal barrier to nonspecific macromolecular absorption. II. Role of dietary corticosterone. *Pediatric Research* **341:** 50–57.

Trier JS (1991) Structure and functions of M cells. *Gastroenterology Clinics of North America* **20:** 531–547.

Udall JN, Pang K, Fritze L et al (1981) Development of gastrointestinal mucosal barrier. I. The effect of age on intestinal permeability to macromolecules. *Pediatric Research* **15:** 241–244.

van Leeuwen PA, Boermeester MA, Houdijk AP et al (1994) Clinical significance of translocation. *Gut* **35 (supplement 1):** S28–S34.

van Voorhis WC, Valinsky J, Hoffman E et al (1983) Relative efficacy of human monocytes and dendritic cells as accessory cells for T cell replication. *Journal of Experimental Medicine* **158:** 174–191.

Wells CL, Jechorek RP, Olmsted SB & Erlandsen SL (1993) Effect on epithelial integrity and bacterial uptake in the polarized human enterocyte-like cell line Caco-2. *Circulatory Shock* **40:** 276–288.

Willems F, Marchant A, Delville JP et al (1994) Interleukin-10 inhibits B7 and intercellular adhesion molecule-1 expression on human monocytes. *European Journal of Immunology* **24:** 1007–1009.

Willman CL, Stewart CC, Miller V et al (1989) Regulation of MHC class II gene expression in macrophages by hematopoetic colony-stimulating factors (CSF). Induction by granulocyte/macrophage CSF and inhibition by CSF-1. *Journal of Experimental Medicine* **170:** 1559–1567.

Wiman K, Curman B, Forsum U et al (1978) Occurrence of Ia antigens on tissues of non-lymphoid origin. *Nature* **276:** 711–713.

Wolf JL, Rubin DH, Finberg R et al (1981) Intestinal M cells: a pathway for entry of reovirus into the host. *Science* **212:** 471.

Zhang ZY & Michael JG (1990) Orally inducible immune unresponsiveness is abrogated by IFN-gamma treatment. *Journal of Immunology* **144:** 4163–4165.

3

Special features of the intestinal lymphocytic system

GEORG KÖHNE
THOMAS SCHNEIDER
MARTIN ZEITZ

The intestinal mucosa has a surface of about 100–400 m². Due to the enormous amount of antigens and mitogens in the gut lumen it is the most important barrier to the external environment. The distinction between a systemic immune response or a tolerance induction towards an antigen is realized by a specialized local immune system termed gut-associated lymphoid tissue (GALT). Two functional compartments can be discerned, an afferent part (Figure 1A), consisting of the organized lymphoid follicles, for example, the Peyer's patches of the ileum, and an effector part (Figure 1B), consisting of the lymphocytes located diffusely in the lamina propria (lamina propria lymphocytes, LPL) and those located above the

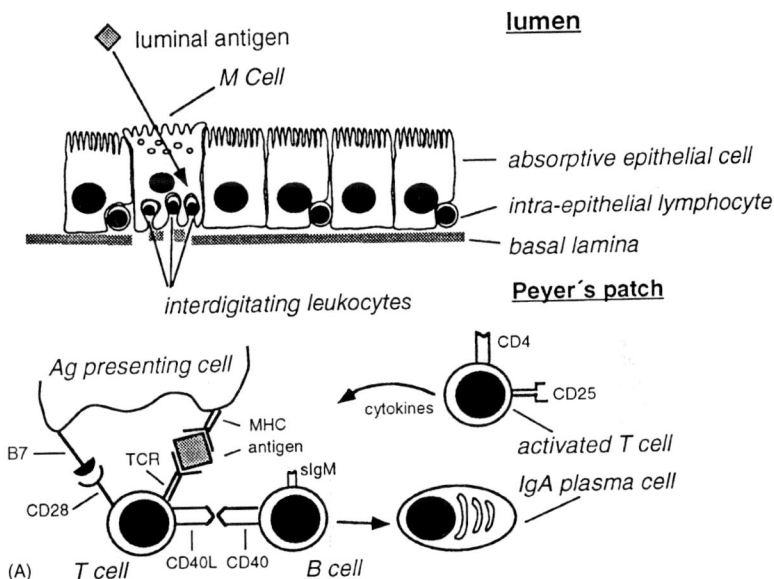

Baillière's Clinical Gastroenterology—
Vol. 10, No. 3, September 1996
ISBN 0–7020–2187–3
0950–3528/96/030427 + 16 $12.00/00

427

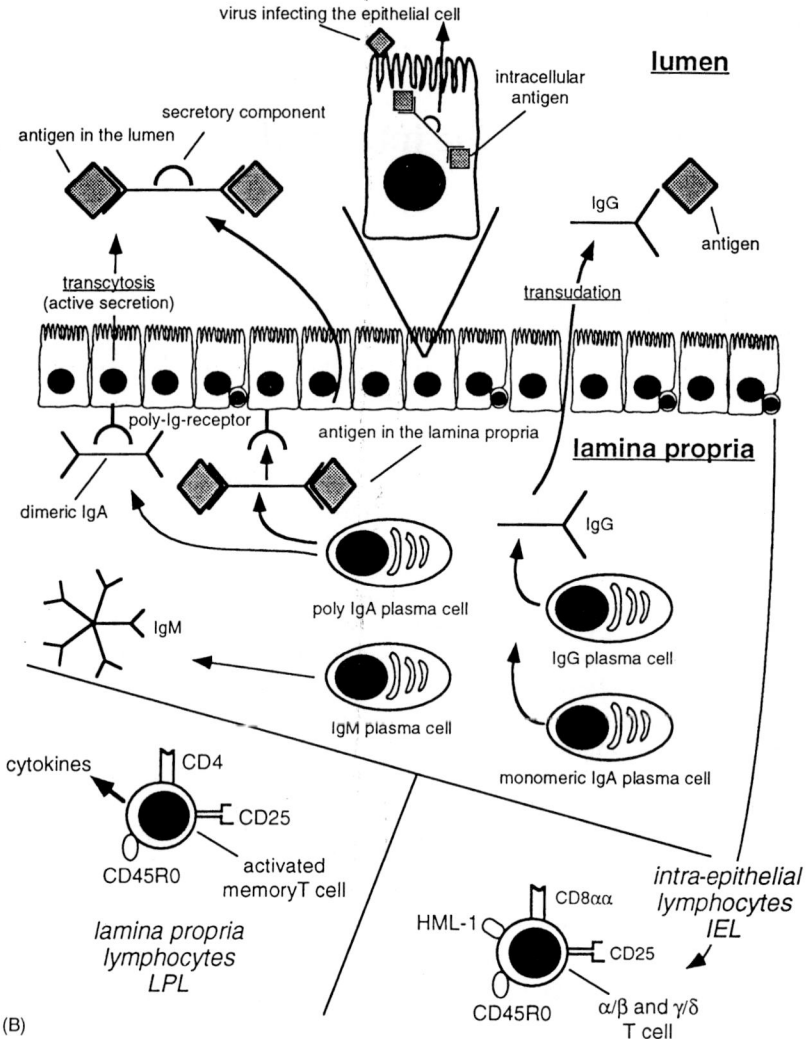

Figure 1. (A) Peyer's patches and the follicle-associated epthelium represent the inductive part of the gastrointestinal immune system. After transport through M cells, which are part of the follicle-associated epithelium, luminal antigens are processed by antigen-presenting cells and presented to T cells in Peyer's patches. These T cells activate precursor B cells which predominantly differentiate to IgA plasma cells. (B) The effector part of the mucosal immune system is dominated by differentiated T cells (IEL and LPL) and the secretory IgA system. T cells are of the activated memory phenotype, proliferate poorly after stimulation of the TCR, and produce large amounts of cytokines. IgA produced by lamina propria plasma cells can bind antigens in the lamina propria, in the epithelial cells and in the gut lumen. Dimeric IgA and pentameric IgM are actively secreted into the lumen after binding to the poly-Ig-receptor and transcytosis by epithelial cells. The major function of mucosal IgA is antigen exclusion. IgG and monomeric IgA are also produced in the mucosa and can reach the lumen by passive paracellular diffusion.

basement membrane between the enterocytes (intra-epithelial lymphocytes, IEL).

It is assumed that antigen enters the intestinal mucosa via the M cells (microfolded cells) which constitute a specialized epithelium above the lymphoid follicles. In these follicles the mucosal immune response is initiated by the uptake and processing of antigenic material by macrophages and follicular dendritic cells and its presentation to T and B cells. Primed lymphocytes leave the mucosa and, after expansion in mesenteric lymph nodes, enter the circulation via the thoracic duct. Finally, they migrate back to the intestinal mucosa—a phenomenon called 'homing'—where they exert their effector functions.

The special features of the phenotype and functional properties of the distinct parts of the gastrointestinal lymphocytic system will be discussed in this review.

M CELLS AND THEIR RELATIONSHIPS TO PEYER'S PATCH LYMPHOCYTES

The organized lymphoid follicles, including the Peyer's patches with the follicle-associated epithelium (FAE) and M cells (microfolded or membranous epthelial cells), are, apart from the mesenteric lymph nodes, the major part of the mucosal inductive site where the immune response is initiated. M cells represent a population of FAE and are most abundant along the upper portion of follicle domes. The FAE is composed mainly of M cells, columnar epithelial cells, IELs, infrequently mucus-secreting goblet cells, and occasional tuft cells. M cells exhibit characteristic ultra-structural features: the layer of glycocalyx and mucus on M cells is quite sparse, compared with that on adjacent columnar cells. They have fewer, shorter and sometimes branched microvilli in contrast to absorptive cells (Owen and Jones, 1974). These very thin (≈ 0.3 mm) parts of the epithelial barrier show numerous apical vesicles; the nucleus is usually located in the basal cytoplasm beneath multiple basal invaginations containing lympho-cytes (including CD4[+] helper cells, CD8[+] suppressor cells, B cells), dentritic cells, and macrophages (Figure 1A). B lymphocytes of the M cell area are phenotypically heterogeneous, whereas T cells predominantly exhibit the CD4[+]CD45RO[+] 'memory' phenotype. T cells of the γ/δ T cell receptor type cannot be detected in M cell areas (Farstad et al, 1993). The origin of M cells remains unclear. It is not yet known whether they derive from trans-formed absorptive cells or develop directly from undifferentiated crypt cells (Bye et al, 1984).

M cells are adapted to uptake and to transport luminal antigens, includ-ing viruses, bacteria and even small parasites (Owen and Jones, 1974; Owen and Nemanic, 1978; Owen et al, 1986). Antigen uptake by M cells usually does not result in degradation, but, instead, in the delivery of the intact antigen into the underlying lymphoid tissue. Thus, these antigens become easily accessible for the interdigitating lymphocytes and macrophages (Bye et al, 1984, Pappo et al, 1991). However, more recently

Allan and co-workers showed that M cells to some degree possess acidic endosomal, prolysosomal, and lysosomal compartments and express MHC class II in these structures (Allan et al, 1993). These data suggest that M cells may have some potential for processing endocytosed antigens and presenting them to immuncompetent cells in their pockets. Furthermore, it has been proposed that M cells provide an opportunity for juxtaposed B lymphocytes to present luminal antigens to adjacent memory T cells (Farstad et al, 1994).

PEYER'S PATCHES

Peyer's patches differ from lymph nodes because they lack afferent lymphatics. Their characteristic feature is that antigen is sampled from the lumen by overlying epithelium, especially by M cells. Patches are most abundant in the terminal ileum. Peyer's patches consist of varying numbers of follicles often with germinal centres and mantle zones of B lymphocytes, interspersed with T cells, predominantly CD4 helper T cells, and macrophages that function as antigen-presenting cells. T cells are numerous in the interfollicular zones and also in the dome areas. CD4 T cells predominate over CD8 T cells in Peyer's patches (Brandtzaeg and Bjerke, 1990). T cell receptor γ/δ-positive cells are quite rare in human Peyer's patches (Farstad et al, 1993). Before lympoblasts can reach FAE to be enfolded within M cells and brought into contact with antigens in Peyer's patches, they must leave the systemic circulation via post-capillary venules. The migration is controlled by surface markers such as the lymphocyte adhesion molecules LECAM-1 and CD44 (see below). Lymphoblasts then enter the follicle-associated epithelium through holes in the basal membrane at the M cell base. Passage to the gut lumen seems to be possible only through the cytoplasm of M cells and does not affect intercellular junctions of the follicle epithelium (Regoli et al, 1994). The efferent lymphatics of Peyer's patches drain to the mesenteric lymph nodes.

INTESTINAL EPITHELIAL CELLS (IEC)

The absorptive cells of the intestinal epithelium also exhibit numerous functions as immune modulation cells. Apart from their function of fluid, electrolyte and nutrient absorption, their role in secretory immunity has been well known for a long time. Dimeric IgA produced in the lamina propria can be transported into the lumen after binding to the secretory component derived from epithelial cells.

More recently IEC have been identified as playing a role in regulating cellular immune responses. It has been demonstrated that IEC constitutively express class II molecules. HLA-DR expression is more prominent in the small bowel than in the colon, HLA-DP expression can be observed at lower levels, and HLA-DQ expression is absent on IEC (Mayer et al, 1991). Since class II molecules are involved in helper T cell activation, IEC are canditate cells for antigen presentation to T cells, especially of the CD4⁺ phenotype. However, it has been shown that IEC preferentially stimulate CD8⁺ suppressor T cells (Bland and Warren, 1986; Mayer and Shlien, 1987). This is in conflict with the well-known class II–CD4⁺ and class I–CD8⁺ interaction. Furthermore, monoclonal antibodies to class I or class II anitigens do not inhibit the lymphocyte stimulation in T cell–epithelial cell interaction (Panja et al, 1994). So it has been proposed that non-classical restriction elements are involved in the stimulation of lympho-cytes by intestinal epithelial cells (Blumberg et al, 1991; Mayer, 1995). CD1 genes are non-polymorphic MHC class I-like molecules. It has been shown that CD1d, which is a member of the CD1 gene family, is involved in T cell–intestinal epithelial cell interactions in a mixed lymphocyte reaction using IEC and peripheral blood T cells. However, this could not be demonstrated for lamina propria T cells (Panja et al, 1993). Other ligands for CD8 have been claimed; the involvement of a 180 kDa glycoprotein (gp180) expressed on IEC has been discussed (Mayer, 1995). Gp180 seems to bind to CD8 and activate an associated *src*-like tyrosine kinase (*src* = the oncogene of Rous sarcoma virus which encodes a non-receptor protein tyrosin kinase). Additionally, apart from the typical protein antigens, epithelial cells have been shown to be able to present exogenous bacterial superantigens, which do not require processing by antigen-presenting cells, and bind to the external domain of the class II major histocompatibility molecule, to mucosal T lymphocytes (Aisenberg et al, 1993).

EXPRESSION OF ADHESION MOLECULES AND CELLULAR TRAFFIC IN THE GALT

Lymphocytes circulate between the bloodstream and various lymphoid tissues. It is generally accepted that the homing of peripheral blood lymphocytes (PBL) into lymphoid tissues such as lymph nodes and Peyer's patches is regulated by interactions with specialized post-capillary venules, especially high endothelial venules (HEVs) (Chin et al, 1991). These interactions display tissue selectivity and are probably determined by a combination of sequential adhesion and activating events during cell–cell and cell–extracellular matrix interactions. Migration of PBL into the lamina propria or the intestinal epithelium is not well established and the molecules involved have to be further determined.

A number of adhesion molecules are involved in lymphocyte homing. These include adhesion molecules of the integrin family, which comprises at least 23 different αβ heterodimers. The β7 integrin group includes two members which are supposed to be involved in lymphocyte homing into mucosal tissues: α4β7 and aᴱβ7 (also called HML-1(human mucosal lymphocyte antigen)) (Cerf-Bensussan et al, 1987; Postigio et al, 1993). Monoclonal antibodies directed against the α4 or β7 integrin-chain inhibit the homing of lymphocytes to mucosal tissues, but not to peripheral lymph nodes (Hamann et al, 1994). Lymphocyte binding to Peyer's patches' HEVs involves the mucosal vascular addressin, MAdCAM-1 (mucosal addressin cell adhesion molecule 1), a member of the IgG and mucin-like families of adhesion receptors with structure homologies to IgA1, which is selectively expressed by venules in mucosal tissues (Briskin et al, 1993). MAdCAM-1 has been shown to bind preferentially to the $\alpha 4\beta 7$ lymphocyte integrin (Berlin et al, 1993). The adhesiveness of Peyer's patch high endothelial venules for lymphocytes can be influenced by cytokines: TNFα, γIFN and IL-4 enhance, and TGF-β down-regulates, lymphocyte binding to HEV (Chin et al, 1992).

HML-1 antigen (CD103) is nearly exclusively expressed in the mucosal immune system, approximately 40% of lamina propria lymphocytes and nearly all IEL are HML-1-positive (Cerf-Bensussan et al, 1987; Ullrich et al, 1990a). HML-1 has also been identified as a member of the integrin family, consisting of a $\beta 7$ subunit associated with a distinctive α-chain (Cerf-Bensussan et al, 1992; Parker et al, 1992). However, in a mouse model, it could not be demonstrated that α^E antigen expression correlates with a distinct homing behaviour (Austrup et al, 1995). Recently, increasing evidence has emerged that HML-1 is predominantly involved in the binding of IEL to enterocytes. It could be demonstrated that the adhesion between epithelial cells and IEL is mediated by the binding of HML-1 to E-cadherin, its ligand on epithelial cells (Cepek et al, 1994). The functional importance of HML-1 for human IEL is further underlined by the observation that the CD3-induced activation of IEL can be enhanced by stimulation of the $\beta 7$-containing integrin (Sarnacki et al, 1992).

The $\beta 2$ integrin family contains three molecules: LFA-1(CD11a/CD18), Mac-1(CD11b/CD18) and p150/95 (CD11c/CD18). These molecules consist of unique α-chains (CD11a–c) and a common β-chain (CD18) and predominantly mediate binding to cellular structures. CD11b+ T cells were rarely observed in LPL in contrast to PBL, which showed approximately 20% CD11b expression (Hoshino et al, 1993). Similarly, CD11a/CD18+ cells were slightly reduced in LPL (Schieferdecker et al, 1992). This is consistent with the finding that LFA-1 is obviously not involved in the homing processes of lymphocytes to the lamina propria (Westermann et al, 1994).

According to other adhesion molecules, IEL exhibit a lower CD11a (LFA-1) (Sarnacki et al, 1991; Ebert, 1993) and CD11b (Hoshino et al, 1993) expression than PBL. CD54 (ICAM-1) and CD58 (LFA-3) were slightly more frequent in IEL than in PBL (Ebert, 1993), and CD29 ($\beta 1$ integrin), which is expressed at high levels by peripheral blood CD45RO+ memory cells, was expressed only in variable percentages and expression was weak (Sarnacki et al, 1991). The expression of LFA-1, HML-1, CD44 was slightly down-regulated, and the expression from ICAM-1 and VLA-4 on human duodenal IEL could be induced by PHA stimulation (Kelleher et al, 1994).

The selective nature of lymphocyte homing to mucosal tissues should not be overemphasized. A number of other adhesion molecules and addressins are involved in homing processes. These include VLA-4, VLA-5, ICAM-1, VCAM, L-selectin or CD44 (Thiele, 1991). Although they are involved generally in homing processes, there is no convincing evidence that they act selectively in the gut (Pabst, 1991; Hamann et al, 1994; Westermann et al, 1994).

Migrating lymphocytes derived from Peyer's patches leave the gut via mesenteric lymph nodes, the lymphatics and the thoracic duct. In the lymphocyte population leaving the gut T cells clearly outnumber B cells. However, in an animal model up to 55% of the IgA$^+$ and 25% of the IgM$^+$ B cells could be identified as newly formed, probably by proliferation in the mucosal wall. On the contrary, only 8.5% of the T cells were derived from recent proliferation in the gut. It is more likely that these T cells originate from Peyer's patches and the interfollicular area than from the lamina propria or the epithelium (Rothkötter et al, 1995).

LAMINA PROPRIA LYMPHOCYTES (LPL)

Mucosal lymphocytes diffusely disseminated in the intestinal lamina propria are termed lamina propria lymphocytes (LPL). They represent a lymphocyte population with functional and phenotypic properties different from other lymphocytic compartments, for example, peripheral blood lymphocytes (PBL), intra-epithelial lymphocytes (IEL) or lymphocytes in organized lymphoid tissues. More than 95% of the LPL express the α/β-type of the T cell receptor (Ullrich et al, 1990a). The proportion of γ/δ T cells in the lamina propria is comparable to the peripheral blood (Table 1) (Ullrich et al, 1990a; Deusch et al, 1991a). The V/δ2-encoded subset predominates the lamina propria γ/δ T cell population (Farstad et al, 1993). CD4$^+$ and CD8$^+$ T cells are present in the lamina propria in a similar proportion compared to the peripheral blood (Selby et al, 1983; James et al, 1986; Schieferdecker et al, 1990). Thus, with respect to the major T cell populations, peripheral blood and lamina propria T cells do not exhibit major differences.

Almost all CD8$^+$ T cells in the adult human intestine express the CD8αβ heterodimer. However, in the fetal intestine almost half of the CD8$^+$ cells in

Table 1. Main phenotypical and functional properties of LPL (lamina propria lymphocytes) and IEL (intra-epithelial lymphocytes) in comparison to PBL (peripheral blood lymphocytes) (for details and references see text).

	LPL	IEL
α/β TCR	↔	↓
γ/δ TCR	↔	↑
CD4	↔	↓↓
CD8	↔	↑↑
CD45RO	↑↑↑	↑↑↑
CD45RA	↓↓	↓↓
HML-1 (α^{E}β7)	↑↑	↑↑↑
CD11a/CD18	↓	↓
CD11b/CD18	↓	↓
CD45RO$^+$/CD29	↓	↓
L-selectin	↓↓	?
CD25	↑↑	↑↑
Proliferation after TCR/CD3 activation	↓↓	↓?
Proliferation after CD2 activation	↑↑↑	?
Cytokine production after TCR/CD3 activation	↑↑↑	?

the lamina propria, but not in Peyer's patches, are positive for the CD8αα homodimer, which is supposed to be a feature of extrathymic T cell maturation (Latthe et al, 1994). So it may be supposed that human lamina propria γ/δ T cells are also partially of extrathymic origin.

One of the first differences found between PBL and LPL indicating maturational differences was the demonstration of a low expression of L-selectin (Leu-8, Mel-14 antigen, LAM-1, LECAM-1) on human and non-human primate lamina propria T cells (Cerf-Bensussan et al, 1985; James et al, 1986, 1987; Kanof et al, 1988; Farstad et al, 1993). L-selectin is a Ca^{2+}-dependent lectin-like receptor that mediates lymphocyte attachment to high endothelial venules of peripheral lymph nodes. Its endothelium-derived ligands GlyCAM-1 and CD34 could not be demonstrated in Peyer's patches in contrast to the expression in peripheral lymph nodes (Kikuta and Rosen, 1994). Additionally, in contrast to PBL, LPL nearly exclusively express the CD45RO antigen (Table 1) (Schieferdecker et al, 1990). Memory T cells are, by definition, cells which have already been in contact with antigen. In the peripheral blood, memory cells express the CD45RO cell-surface glycoprotein complex and CD29, the β1-chain of the integrin family (Sanders et al, 1988). Thus, when looking at CD45 expression, the phenotype of LPL resembles that of memory T cells. However, lamina propria memory cells do not share all characteristics of peripheral memory T cells. CD29 (β1 integrin) is a member of the integrin family of adhesion molecules which seem to be predominantly involved in the recognition of components of the extracellular matrix. In contrast to peripheral blood CD45RO⁺ memory cells, lamina propria memory cells had reduced percentages of CD29⁺ cells (Schieferdecker et al, 1992).

The balance between memory cells and unprimed CD4 T cells seems to be very important for the immunoregulation in the gut since the transfer of CD45RB^hi memory cells to athymic nude mice results in severe intestinal inflammation. The disease can be prevented if CD45RB^lo virgin cells are co-transfected to these mice (Morrissey and Charrier, 1995).

In humans, approximately 40% of the LPL express the surface antigen recognized by HML-1 (α^Eβ7), whereas only a few (~2%) peripheral T cells are HML-1⁺ (Cerf-Bensussan et al, 1987; Schieferdecker et al, 1990, 1992). Dual colour cytofluorometry has shown that HML-1 is preferentially expressed on CD8⁺ T cells; however, a significant proportion of CD4⁺ lamina propria T cells also express HML-1 (Schieferdecker et al, 1990). The low number of CD45RA⁺ cells in the human intestinal lamina propria is almost exclusively HML-1⁻. It has therefore been hypothesized that HML-1 may be a tissue-specific memory T cell marker exclusively expressed in the environment of the gut (Schieferdecker et al, 1991). The potential role of HML-1 as a homing and adhesion molecule has already been discussed above. Furthermore, expression of HML-1 can be induced on HML-1⁻ PBL by in vitro activation, so it was proposed that HML-1 is an activation marker (Schieferdecker et al, 1990).

Additionally, lamina propria T cells have been found to express other activation markers. The expression of the IL-2 receptor and the synthesis of IL-2 by T cells are central events in the initiation and regulation of antigen-

or mitogen-induced immune responses (Smith, 1988). Using Northern blot analysis in non-human primates to study the transcription of the gene for the IL-2 receptor α-chain (CD25), it has been shown that mRNA for the IL-2 receptor α-chain is clearly detectable in freshly isolated lymphocytes from the intestinal lamina propria, whereas in the other populations from the spleen, mesenteric lymph nodes, or the peripheral blood, IL-2 receptor mRNA is found only after activation in vitro (Zeitz et al, 1988a). Correspondingly, the proportion of intestinal LPL expressing CD25 is higher than that of PBL (Table 1). The increased CD25 expression of LPL is correlated with a high proliferative response to low doses of IL-2, indicating that the IL-2 receptors are able to transduce the signal after IL-2 binding. In agreement with an increased state of activation of lamina propria T cells, these cells are able to synthesize large amounts of IL-2 after activation (Zeitz et al, 1988a).

CD69 is a 28–32 kDa disulphide-linked homodimer expressed very quickly and transiently upon TCR/CD3 cross-linking in T cells. It therefore represents another useful marker for recent T cell activation. Expression of CD69 was found on 80–90% of CD4+, 90–100% of CD8+ and all γ/δ lamina propria T cells, and was virtually absent on peripheral T cells (DeMaria et al, 1993). Thus, CD69 can be regarded as another T cell activation marker preferentially expressed in the intestinal mucosa. LPL also express major histocompatibility complex (MHC) class II antigens (Zeitz et al, 1988a) and other T cell activation markers (Peters et al, 1986).

The continuous activation state of LPL cannot only be observed by studying the phenotype. LPL have significantly higher basal intracytoplasmic Ca^{2+} levels compared with autologous PBL (DeMaria et al, 1993). This was reversible after 24 hours of culture in pure medium, which points to a special importance of the intestinal micro-environment. The increased state of activation of lamina propria T cells may be the result of the permanent exposure to antigens and mitogens in the gut lumen.

LPL, whose phenotype resembles that of memory T cells, show a distinct behaviour on exposure to recall antigens. While PBL, lymphocytes from the spleen, and mesenteric lymph node of non-human primates immunized by rectal mucosal injection of *Chlamydia trachomatis* show a clear proliferative response to the recall antigen *Chlamydia trachomatis*, LPL do not proliferate (Zeitz et al, 1988b). This was not due to the absence of antigen-reactive T cells in the intestinal lamina propria because these T cells provided helper function for immunglobulin synthesis by spleen B cells. Additionally, it was demonstrated that the antigen receptor-(TCR/CD3)-dependent activation pathway in lamina propria T cells is down-regulated. In contrast, responsiveness to CD2 and CD28 stimulation seems to be preserved (Pirzer et al, 1990). After CD2 ligation LPL were even more responsive than PBL, as determined by release of cytokines. The CD2>CD3 dominance in γIFN, IL-2, IL-4, and TNFα release could be exaggerated by CD28 co-ligation (Targan et al, 1995). It has been proposed that changes in the CD2 post-receptor pathway are involved in these phenomena. Co-culture of PBL with intestinal mucosa supernatants can lead to a functional behaviour similar to that found in freshly isolated LPL.

Small, non-protein, non-peptide molecules with oxidative properties have been proposed to mediate this down-regulation of CD3-induced T cell proliferation (Qiao et al, 1993).

INTRA-EPITHELIAL LYMPHOCYTES (IEL)

Intra-epithelial lymphocytes reside between intestinal epithelial cells near the basement membrane and represent a large population of lymphocytes located at the interface between the body and the antigenic intestinal microflora. Because of this extraordinary location at the frontier of the gastrointestinal immune system they are strong candidates for carrying out specialized functions with regard to the epithelial barrier system.

Phenotypically, IEL exhibit distinct features. Intra-epithelial T lymphocytes are, in contrast to lamina propria and PBL, mainly CD8$^+$ (~70%), and they express the γ/δ T cell receptor in a higher proportion (Table 1) (Ullrich et al, 1990a; Deusch et al, 1991a). In human colonic epithelium, γ/δ T cell receptor-expressing lymphocytes predominantly use the Vδ1 gene segment, which was attributed to a preferential homing or a local expansion of these cells (Deusch et al, 1991b; Farstad et al, 1993). Lamina propria and Peyer's patch γ/δ T cells preferentially express the Vδ2 gene product, so it seems unlikely that γ/δ T cells of the human epithelium originate from these compartments (Farstad et al, 1993). Apart from the limited Vδ usage, the oligoclonality of IEL is further underlined by a limited Vβ gene segment usage of the $\alpha\beta$ T cell receptor (Kerckhove et al, 1992; Plüschke et al, 1994).

The most striking phenotypical feature of IEL may be that almost all IEL are HML-1($\alpha^E\beta7$)$^+$ (Table 1) (Cerf-Bensussan et al, 1987; Ullrich et al, 1990a). Furthermore, like LPL, IEL express activation and memory cell type markers (Table 1) (Ullrich et al, 1990a; Sarnacki et al, 1991; Ebert, 1993).

According to the NK (natural killer) cell markers CD16/CD56, another specific difference of the IEL fraction is that the double positive fraction (~40%) of CD3$^+$/CD16$^+$/CD56$^+$ T cells is much higher than that observed in LPL or PBL (9 and 6%, respectively). This difference was due to a 10-fold increase in expression of the CD16 molecule (Deusch et al, 1991b). Others reported a spontaneous cytotoxicity or natural killer activity of human IEL, which could be inhibited by HML-1 (a$^E\beta7$ integrin) antibody treatment (Cerf-Bensussan et al, 1985; Taunk et al, 1992; Roberts et al, 1993).

In experimental models using cultured epithelial monolayers and a mucosal derived T lymphocyte cell line it was demonstrated that lymphocytes can dramatically alter the profile of epithelial surface functions, for example, a decreased monolayer resistance and decreased epithelial electrogenic Cl$^-$ secretion (Kaoutzani et al, 1994). This points to a close inter-relationship between IEL and epithelial cells with respect to the epithelial barrier function in the gut.

The results concerning the proliferative properties of human IEL are controversial. For instance, a low proliferative capacity of human IEL to T cell stimuli has been reported (Ebert et al, 1989), whereas others described a similar proliferative response of IEL and PBL enriched in CD8[+] cells to optimal concentrations of immobilized OKT3 (Sarnacki et al, 1992).

Another function of IEL is their suppressor cell activity. For example, IEL down-regulate the proliferative response of primed allogenic peripheral bood mononuclear cells. This suppressor function seems to be important for effective mucosal immune regulation (Dalton et al, 1993).

On the basis of studies in mice, where there is increasing evidence for extrathymic T cell maturation in the intestinal epithelium (simultaneous expression of CD4 and CD8, expression of the CD8αα homodimer and detection of RAG1 RNA, reviewed in Lynch et al (1995)), it has been proposed that the epithelium of the human intestine may be a site of extrathymic T cell maturation. Recently, RAG (recombination activation gene) expression could be detected in the human intestinal epithelium using RT-PCR (Lynch et al, 1995). Expression of the RAG genes is associated with TCR gene rearrangement in the thymus, and expression ceases once rearrangement is complete. Additionally, CD8αα homodimer-bearing T cells could be identified in human lamina propria and epithelium in human fetal intestine (Latthe et al, 1994). Furthermore, the fraction of CD5[+] γ/δ T cells in the human epithelium was much lower than in PBL (Deusch et al, 1991b). Expression of CD5 on the surface of peripheral blood T lymphocytes is believed to indicate their thymic origin. Taken together, there are increasing data which support the hypothesis that the human epithelium is a site of extrathymic T cell maturation.

MUCOSAL HUMORAL IMMUNE MECHANISMS

One major well-known defence mechanism in the gut is the IgA system as part of the mucosal humoral immune system. In contrast to circulating B cells, or rather plasma cells, which secrete mainly IgG and IgM, mucosal plasma cells produce predominantly IgA. Among the immunoglobulin isotypes present on mucosal surfaces as a result of active secretion (di- and polymeric IgA, polymeric IgM) or of transudation (IgG, monomeric IgA), secretory IgA (sIgA) is particularly stable and well suited to function in the enzymatically hostile environment of the gastrointestinal tract. This stability is achieved largely by the secretory component (SC) which makes secretory IgA less susceptible to attack by metabolic and microbial enzymes (Brown et al, 1970; Weiker and Underdown, 1975; Brandtzaeg, 1981). In contrast to sIgM, the complex of polymeric IgA and SC is stabilized by covalent linkages which may enhance resistance to enzymes. Moreover, sIgA has been shown to bind trypsin and chymotrypsin in an antibody-independent manner that inactivates these enzymes (Shim et al, 1969).

The synthesis of IgA is highly dependent on activated CD4[+] T cells. In the interaction between the activated CD4[+] T cell and the B cell a pair of accessory molecules (CD4OL/CD40) play a crucial role for the initiation of Ig heavy-chain constant-region (C_H) gene switching. Cytokines produced mainly by activated T lymphocytes (e.g. transforming growth factor β

(TGFβ), interleukin 2 (IL-2), IL-5, IL-6, and IL-10) have been identified in experimental animals as important cytokines for clonal expansion of activated B cells and the switch from IgM to IgA production (Strober and Ehrhardt, 1994) (Figure 1A).

The main function of secretory antibodies is immune exclusion (Stokes et al, 1975). This term was introduced for mechanisms which keep micro-organisms, bacterial toxins, viruses and other potentially harmful antigenic material out of the interior of the body (Figure 1B). Recently, additional roles for IgA in the mucosal defence, contributing to immune exclusion, have been recognized (Mazanec et al, 1993). The majority of the mucosal IgA enters the intestinal lumen via epithelial transcytosis mediated by the polymeric Ig receptor (Figure 1B). Besides its function of blocking the adherence of agents to the epthelial cells, secretory IgA is also capable of inhibiting virus assembly intracellularly and virus release from epithelial cells (Mazanec et al, 1992). This may occur when a transcytotic vesicle containing anti-viral IgA fuses with an exocytotic vesicle from the Golgi that contains viral glycoproteins. Furthermore, secretory IgA may also bind to an agent in the lamina propria which is consecutively eliminated by transcytosis of the immune complex through the epthelial cell into the lumen (Figure 1B) (Kaetzel et al, 1991).

Because IgA antibodies lack ordinary complement-activating properties (Russell and Mansa, 1989), immune exclusion is principally a non-inflammatory mechanism. The cellular basis for this 'first-line specific defence' is that exocrine glands and secretory mucosa contain most of the body's activated B cells, particularly the gut lamina propria, where at least 80% of all Ig-producing immunocytes (B-cell blasts and plasma cells) are found (Brandtzaeg et al, 1989). More sIgA is, in fact, secreted every day into the intestinal lumen than the total daily production of IgG in the peripheral blood (Conley and Delacroix, 1987). The intestinal mucosa is therefore a major effector site of specific immune response and offers the possibility of activation by oral immunization. Thus, potent vaccines against different pathogens may be gained in the future.

SUMMARY

The gastrointestinal lymphocytic system can be divided in two functional compartments, the organized lymphoid tissue, for example, the Peyer's patches, and the lymphocytes located diffusely in the mucosa, the lamina propria lymphocytes (LPL), and the intra-epithelial lymphocytes (IEL). Antigens enter the Peyer's patches as the afferent part of the GALT via specialized epithelial cells called M cells. After the initiation of the immune response by antigen processing and presentation to B and T cells in Peyer's patches, primed lymphocytes leave the mucosa via the thoracic duct. Finally they migrate back to the mucosa where they exert effector functions. Adhesion molecules, including integrins, especially α4β7 and $\alpha^E\beta7$ (HML-1) are involved in these homing and adhesion processes. LPL and IEL differ from peripheral blood lymphocytes in their expression of adhesion molecules and other surface and activation markers. Additionally, they exhibit functional features different from those of other lymphocyte compartments. In the mucosal immune system, plasma cells mainly secrete IgA, which is part of the specialized humoral defence in the gut.

Acknowledgement

Our studies were supported by grants (FKZ) II-008-91 and (FKZ) 01 KI 9468 from the BMBF and Ze188/4 from the DFG.

REFERENCES

Aisenberg J, Ebert EC & Mayer L (1993) T cell activation in human intestinal mucosa: the role of superantigens. *Gastroenterology* **105:** 1421–1430.

Allan H, Mendrick DL & Trier JS (1993) Rat intestinal M cells contain acidic endosomal-lysosomal compartments and express class II major histocompatibility complex determinants. *Gastroenterology* **104:** 698–708.

Austrup F, Rebstock S, Kilshaw P & Hamann A (1995) Transforming growth factor-beta 1-induced expression of the mucosa-related integrin alpha E on lymphocytes is not associated with mucosa-specific homing. *European Journal of Immunology* **25:** 1487–1491.

Berlin C, Berg EL, Briskin MJ et al (1993) α4β7 Integrin mediates lymphocyte binding to mucosal vascular addressin MAdCAM-1. *Cell* **74:** 185–195.

Bland PW & Warren LG (1986) Antigen presentation by epithelial cells of rat small intestine. I. Selective induction of suppressor T cells. *Immunology* **58:** 9–14.

Blumberg RS, Terhorst C, Bleicher P et al (1991) Expression of a nonpolymorphic MHC class I-like molecule, CD1d, by human intestinal epithelial cells. *Journal of Immunology* **147:** 2518–2524.

Brandtzaeg P (1981) Transport models for secretory IgA and secretory IgM. *Clinical and Experimental Immunology* **44:** 221–232.

Brandtzaeg P & Bjerke K (1990) Immunomorphological characteristics of human Peyer's patches. *Digestion* **46 (supplement 2):** 262–273.

Brandtzaeg P, Halstensen TS, Kett K et al (1989) Immunobiology and immunopathology of human gut mucosa: humoral immunity and IEL. *Gastroenterology* **97:** 1562–1584.

Briskin MJ, McEvoy LM & Butcher EC (1993) The mucosal vascular addressin, MAdCAM-1, displays homology to immunoglobin and mucin-like adhesion receptors and to IgA. *Nature* **363:** 461–464.

Brown WR, Newcomb RW & Ishizaka K (1970) Proteolytic degradation of exocrine and serum immunoglobulin. *Journal of Clinical Investigation* **49:** 1374–1380.

Bye WA, Allan CH & Trier JS (1984) Structure, distribution and origin of M cells in Peyer's patches of mouse ileum. *Gastroenterology* **86:** 789–801.

Cepek K, Shaw S, Parker C et al (1994) Adhesion between epithelial cells and T lymphocytes mediated by E-cadherin and the alpha E beta 7 integrin. *Nature* **372:** 190–193.

Cerf-Bensussan N, Guy-Grand D & Griscelli C (1985) Intraepithelial lymphocytes of human gut: isolation, characterization and study of natural killer activity. *Gut* **26:** 81–88.

Cerf-Bensussan N, Jarry A, Brousse N et al (1987) A monoclonal antibody (HML-1) defining a novel membrane molecule present on human intestinal lymphocytes. *European Journal of Immunology* **17:** 1279–1285.

Cerf-Bensussan N, Begue B, Gagnon J, Meo T (1992) The human intraepithelial lymphocyte marker HML-1 is an integrin consisting of a beta 7 subunit associated with a distinctive alpha chain. *European Journal of Immunology* **22:** 273–277.

Chin Y-H, Cai J-P & Hieselaar T (1991) Lymphocyte migration into mucosal tissues: mechanism and modulation. *Immunologic Research* **10:** 271–278.

Chin Y-H, Cai J-P & Xu X-M (1992) Transforming growth factor-β1 and IL-4 regulate the adhesiveness of Peyer's patch high endothelial venule cells for lymphocytes. *Journal of Immunology* **148:** 1106–1112.

Conley ME & Delacroix DL (1987) Intravascular and mucosal immunoglobulin A: two seperate but related systems of immune defense? *Annals of Internal Medicine* **106:** 892–899.

Dalton HR, Dipaolo MC, Sachdev GK et al (1993) Human colonic intraepithelial lymphocytes from patients with inflammatory bowel disease fail to down-regulate proliferative responses of primed allogenic peripheral blood mononuclear cells after rechallenge with antigens. *Clinical and Experimental Immunology* **93:** 97–102.

DeMaria R, Fais S, Silvestri M et al (1993) Continuous in vivo activation and transient hypo-responsiveness of TCR/CD3 triggering of human lamina propria lymphocytes. *European Journal of Immunology* **23:** 3104–3108.

Deusch K, Lüling F, Reich K et al (1991a) A major fraction of human intraepithelial lymphocytes simultaneously express the gamma/delta T cell receptor, the CD8 accessory molecule and preferentially use the V delta 1 gene segment. *European Journal of Immunology* **21:** 1053–1059.

Deusch K, Pfeffer K, Reich K et al (1991b) Phenotypic and functional characterization of human TCRγ/δ+ intestinal intraepithelial lymphocytes. *Current Topics in Microbiology and Immunology* **173:** 279–283.

Ebert EC (1993) Do the CD45RO⁺CD8⁺ intestinal intraepithelial lymphocytes have the characteristics of memory cells? *Cellular Immunology* **147:** 331–340

Ebert EC, Roberts AI, Brolin RE & Raska K (1989) Examination of the low proliferative capacity of human intraepithelial lymphocytes to various T cell stimuli. *Gastroenterology* **97:** 1372–1381.

Farstad IN, Halstensen TS, Fausa O & Brandtzaeg P (1993) Do human Peyer's patches contribute to the intestinal intraepithelial gamma/delta T-cell-population. *Scandinavian Journal of Immunology* **38:** 451–458.

Farstad IN, Haltensen TS, Fausa O & Brandtzaeg P (1994) Heterogeneity of M-cell-associated B and T cells in human Peyer's patches. *Immunology* **83:** 457–464.

Hamann A, Andrew DP, Jablonski-Westrich D et al (1994) Role of α4-integrins in lymphocyte homing to mucosal tissues in vivo. *Journal of Immunology* **152:** 3282–3293.

Hoshino T, Yamada A, Honda J et al (1993) Tissue-specific distribution and age dependent increase of human CD11b⁺ T cells. *Journal of Immunology* **151:** 2237–2246.

James SP, Fiocchi C, Graeff AS & Strober W (1986) Phenotypic analysis of lamina propria lympho-cytes. Predominance of helper-inducer and cytolytic T-cell phenotypes in Crohn's disease and control patients. *Gastroenterology* **91:** 1483–1489.

James SP, Graeff AS & Zeitz M (1987) Predominance of the helper-inducer T cells in mesenteric lymph nodes and intestinal lamina propria of normal nonhuman primates. *Cellular Immunology* **107:** 372–383.

Kaetzel CS, Robinson JK, Chintalacharuvu KR et al (1991) The polymeric immunoglobulin receptor (secretory component) mediates transport of immune complexes across epithelial cells: a local defense function for IgA. *Proceedings of the National Academy of Sciences of the USA* **88:** 8796–8800.

Kanof ME, Strober W, Fiocchi C et al (1988) CD4 positive Leu-8 negative helper-inducer T cells predominate in the human lamina propria. *Journal of Immunology* **141:** 3029–3036.

Kaoutzani P, Colgan SP, Cepek KL et al (1994) Reconstitution of cultured epithelial monolayers with a mucosal derived T lymphocyte cell line. *Journal of Clinical Investigation* **94:** 788–796.

Kelleher D, Murphy A, Lynch S & O'Farrely C (1994) Adhesion molecules utilized in binding of intraepithelial lymphocytes to human enterocytes. *European Journal of Immunology* **24:** 1013–1016.

Kerckhove CV, Russel GJ, Deusch K et al (1992) Oligoclonality of human intestinal intraepithelial T cells. *Journal of Experimental Medicine* **175:** 57–63

Kikuta A & Rosen SD (1994) Localisation of ligands for L-selectin in mouse peripheral lymph node high endothelial cells by colloidal gold conjugates. *Blood* **84:** 3766–3775.

Latthe M, Terry L & MacDonald TT (1994) High frequency of CDαα homodimer-bearing T cells in human fetal intestine. *European Journal of Immunology* **24:** 1703–1705.

Lynch S, Kelleher D, Manus RM & O'Farrelly C (1995) RAG1 and RAG2 expression of human intestinal epithelium: evidence of extrathymic T cell differentiation. *European Journal of Immunology* **25:** 1143–1147.

Mayer L (1995) Intestinal epithelium: a new immunological barrier. In Tytgat GNJ, Bartelsman JFWM & van Deventer SJH (eds) *Falk Symposium 85, Inflammatory Bowel Diseases*, pp 384–387. Dordrecht: Kluwer Academic Publishers.

Mayer L & Shlien R (1987) Evidence for function of Ia molecule on gut epithelial cells in man. *Journal of Experimental Medicine* **166:** 1471.

Mayer L, Eisenhardt D, Salomon P et al (1991) Expression of class II molecules on intestinal epithelial cells in humans. *Gastroenterology* **100:** 3–12

Mazanec MB, Kaetzel CS, Lamm ME et al (1992) Intracellular neutralization of virus by immunoglobulin A antibodies. *Proceedings of the National Academy of Sciences of the USA* **89:** 6901–6905.
Mazanec MB, Nedrud JG, Kaetzel CS & Lamm ME (1993) A three tiered view of the role of IgA in mucosal defense. *Immunology Today* **14:** 430–435.
Morrissey PJ & Charrier K (1995) Induction of colitis in SCID mice by the transfer of normal CD4⁺/CD45RBhiT cells. In Tytgat GNJ, Bartelsman JFWM & van Deventer SJH (eds) *Falk Symposium 85, Inflammatory Bowel Diseases*, pp 418–423. Dordrecht: Kluwer Academic Publishers.
Owen RL & Jones AL (1974) Epithelial cell specialization within human Peyer's patch: an ultrastructural study of intestinal lymphoid follicles. *Gastroenterology* **66:** 189–203.
Owen RL & Nemanic P (1978) Antigen processing structures of the mammalian intestinal tract: an SEM study of lymphoepithelial organs. *Scanning Electron Microscopy* **2:** 367–378.
Owen RL, Pierce NF, Apple RT & Gray WC (1986) M cell transport of *Vibrio cholerae* from the intestinal lumen into Peyer's patches: a mechanism for antigen sampling and for microbial transepithelial migration. *Journal of Infectious Diseases* **153:** 1108–1118.
Pabst R (1991) Lymphocyte migration to the gut: oversimplification and controversial aspects. *Immunological Research* **10:** 279–281.
Panja A, Blumberg RS, Balk SP & Mayer L (1993) Cd1d is involved in T cell–intestinal epithelial cell interaction. *Journal of Experimental Medicine* **178:** 1115–1119.
Panja A, Barone A & Mayer L (1994) Stimulation of lamina propria lymphocytes by intestinal epithelial cells: evidence for recognition of nonclassical restriction elements. *Journal of Experimental Medicine* **179:** 943–950.
Pappo J, Ermark TH & Steger HJ (1991) Monoclonal antibody-directed of fluorescent polystyrene microspheres to Peyer's patch M cells. *Immunology* **73:** 277–280.
Parker CM, Cepek KL, Russel GL et al (1992) A family of beta 7 integrins on human mucosal lymphocytes. *Proceedings of the National Academy of Sciences of the USA* **89:** 1924–1928.
Peters M, Secrist H, Anders KR et al (1986) Increased expression of cell surface activation markers by intestinal monunuclear cells. *Clinical Research* **35:** 462–464.
Pirzer UC, Schürmann G, Post S et al (1990) Differential responsiveness to CD3-Ti vs CD2-dependent activation in human intestinal T lymphocytes. *European Journal of Immunology* **20:** 2339–2342.
Plüschke G, Taube H, Krawinkel U et al (1994) Oligoclonality and skewed T cell receptor V beta gene segment expression in in vivo activated human intestinal intraepithelial T lymphocytes. *Immunobiology* **192:** 77–93.
Postigo AA, Sánchez-Mateos P, Lazarovits Al et al (1993) α4β7 Integrin mediates B cell binding to fibronectin and vascular cell adhesion molecule-1. *Journal of Immunology* **151:** 2471–2483.
Qiao L, Schürmann G, Autschbach F et al (1993) Human intestinal mucosa alters T cell reactivities. *Gastroenterology* **105:** 814–819.
Regoli M, Borghesi C, Bertelli E & Nicoletti C (1994) A morphological study of the lymphocyte traffic in Peyer's Patches after in vivo antigenic stimulation. *Anatomical Record* **239:** 47–54.
Roberts AI, O'Connel M, Biancone L et al (1993) Spontaneous cytotoxicity of intestinal intraepithelial lymphocytes: clues to mechanism. *Clinical and Experimental Immunology* **94:** 527–532.
Rothkötter HJ, Hriesik C & Pabst R (1995) More newly formed T than B lymphocytes leave the intestinal mucosa via lymphatics. *European Journal of Immunology* **25:** 886–869.
Russell MW & Mansa B (1989) Complement-fixing properties of human IgA antibodies: alternative pathway complement activation by plastic-bound, but not by specific antigen-bound IgA. *Scandinavian Journal of Immunology* **30:** 175–183.
Sanders ME, Makgoba MW, Sharrow SO et al (1988) Human memory T lymphocytes express increased levels of three cell adhesion molecules (LFA-3, CD2, and LFA-1) and three other molecules (UCHL-1, CDw29, and Pgp-1) and have enhanced IFN-γ production. *Journal of Immunology* **140:** 1401–1407.
Sarnacki S, Bègue B, Jarry A & Cerf-Bensussan N (1991) Human intestinal intraepithelial lymphocytes, a distinct population of activated T cells. *Immunological Research* **10:** 302–305.
Sarnacki S, Bègue B, Buc H et al (1992) Enhancement of CD3-induced activation of human intestinal intraepithelial lymphocytes by stimulation of the β7-containing integrin defined by HML-1 monoclonal antibody. *European Journal of Immunology* **22:** 2887–2892.
Schieferdecker HL, Ullrich R, Weiß-Breckwoldt AN et al (1990) The HML-1 antigen of intestinal lymphocytes is an activation antigen. *Journal of Immunology* **144:** 2541–2549.

Schieferdecker HL, Ullrich R & Zeitz M (1991) Phenotype of HML-1-positive T cells in the human intestinal lamina propria. *Immunulogic Research* **10:** 207–210.

Schieferdecker HL, Ullrich R, Hirseland H & Zeitz M (1992) T cell differentiation antigens on lymphocytes in the human intestinal lamina propria. *Journal of Immunology* **149:** 2816–2822.

Selby WS, Janossy G, Bofill M & Jewell DP (1983) Lymphocyte subpopulations in the human small intestine. The findings in normal mucosa and in the mucosa of patients with adult coeliac disease. *Clinical and Experimental Immunology* **52:** 219–228.

Shim B, Kang YS, Kim WJ et al (1969) Self-protective activity of colostral IgA against tryptic digestion. *Nature* **222:** 787–788.

Smith KA (1988) Interleukin-2, inception, impact, and implications. *Science* **240:** 1169–1176.

Stokes CR, Soothill JF & Turner MW (1975) Immune exclusion is a function of IgA. *Nature* **255:** 745–746.

Strober W & Ehrhardt RO (1994) Regulation of IgA B cell development. In Ogra P, Mestecky R, Lamm ME et al (eds) *Handbook of Mucosal Immunology*, pp 159–176. Orlando, FL: Academic Press.

Targan SR, Deem RL, Liu M et al (1995) Definition of lamina propria T cell responsive state, enhanced cytokine responsiveness of T cells stimulated through the CD2 pathway. *Journal of Immunology* **154:** 664–675.

Taunk J, Roberts AI & Ebert EC (1992) Spontaneous cytotoxicity of human intraepithelial lymphocytes against epithelial cell tumors. *Gastroenterology* **102:** 69–75.

Thiele H-G (1991) Lymphocyte homing: an overview. *Immunological Research* **10:** 261–267.

Ullrich R, Schieferdecker HL, Ziegler K et al (1990a) $\gamma\delta$ T cells in the human intestine express surface markers of activation and are preferentially located in the epithelium. *Cellular Immunology* **128:** 619–627.

Ullrich R, Zeitz M, Heise W et al (1990b) Mucosal atrophy is associated with loss of activated T cells in the duodenal mucosa of human immunodeficiency virus (HIV)-infected patients. *Digestion* **46** **(supplement 2):** 302–307.

Weiker J & Underdown BJ (1975) Secretory component bonding to immunoglobulins A and M. *Journal of Immunology* **114:** 1337–1344.

Westermann J, Nagahori Y, Walter S et al (1994) B and T lymphocyte subsets enter peripheral lymph nodes and Peyer's patches without preference in vivo: no correlation occurs between their localization in different types of high endothelial venules and the expression of CD44, VLA-4, LFA-1, ICAM-1, CD2 or L-selectin. *European Journal of Immunology* **24:** 2312–2316.

Zeitz M, Greene WC, Pfeffer NJ & James SP (1988a) Lymphocytes isolated from the intestinal Lamina propria of normal nonhuman primates have increased expression of genes associated with T-cell activation. *Gastroenterology* **94:** 647–655.

Zeitz M, Quinn TC & Graeff AS (1988b) Mucosal T cells provide helper function but do not proliferate when stimulated by specific antigen in lymphogranuloma venerum proctitis in nonhuman primates. *Gastroenterology* **94:** 353–366.

4

Mucosal allergy: role of mast cells and eosinophil granulocytes in the gut

STEPHAN C. BISCHOFF

THE INTESTINAL BARRIER: PREDESTINED FOR HYPERSENSITIVITY REACTIONS?

The clinical significance of allergic reactions in the gastrointestinal (GI) tract has been an issue of controversy for many years, possibly due to the lack of a clear definition of intestinal allergic disease, the few epidemiological data available, particularly in adults, and the limited knowledge about underlying mechanisms (Farah et al, 1985; Ferguson, 1990; Shanahan, 1993). However, several lines of evidence indicate that allergic reactions may occur not only in the skin and the respiratory mucosa, but also in the GI tract (Crowe and Perdue, 1992; Sampson et al, 1992). The intestinal mucosa must balance two major and largely exclusive functions: nutritional uptake and host defence. To achieve these functions, it is supplied with epithelial cells which form an enormous luminal surface and which are specialized to provide resorption and digestion of nutrients. On the other hand, this characteristic makes the intestinal tract susceptible to foreign antigens in the gut lumen, which contains large quantities of food proteins, microbiological antigens, toxic reagents and even inhalative particles, such as pollens swallowed under normal conditions. Therefore the intestinal mucosa is supplied with a complex defence system consisting of a mucus layer, an epithelial barrier and a network of immunocompetent cells, inflammatory cells, nerves and blood vessels in the lamina propria and submucosa. The discovery and understanding of the regulatory mechanisms has raised the concept of the 'intestinal barrier', which plays a fundamental role in host defence and disease (Brandtzaeg et al, 1989; Fantry and James, 1994). Any dysregulation of the intestinal homeostasis may lead to an increased influx of pathogenic antigens and/or an abnormal immune response, causing inflammatory reactions and diseases such as bacterial infections, intestinal parasitosis or inflammatory bowel diseases. Inflammatory cells mediating intestinal inflammation are either constitutively present in the intestinal tissue (monocytes, eosinophils, mast cells) or migrate from the circulation to the sites of intestinal inflammation (neutrophils, basophils). Thus, the immunological components required to

Baillière's Clinical Gastroenterology—
Vol. 10, No. 3, September 1996
ISBN 0–7020–2187–3
0950–3528/96/030443 + 17 $12.00/00

443

develop an allergic reaction (mast cells, eosinophils, lymphocytes), and potential allergens such as food proteins, are present in large amounts at the intestinal barrier (Crowe and Perdue, 1992). Therefore, as in the case of the respiratory mucosa, which has been studied more extensively in this respect, the intestinal mucosa is predestined for hypersensitivity reactions against foreign antigens.

BASIC MECHANISMS OF ALLERGIC INFLAMMATION

Two phases of IgE-mediated allergic reactions can be distinguished: the sensitization phase, characterized by the induction of specific IgE against particular antigens in genetically predisposed individuals, and the effector phase, which often occurs many years later. The effector phase is initiated by exposure to antigen, which induces an inflammatory reaction consisting of an immediate and a late-phase reaction (Metzger et al, 1985; Charlesworth et al, 1989). The immediate phase is mediated mainly by tissue mast cells which release mediators in response to cross-linking of surface-bound IgE by antigen. The mediators, for example, histamine and leukotrienes, cause an increase in vascular permeability, muscle contraction, oedema, and finally the typical symptoms of immediate allergic reactions such as itching, and weal and flare reactions in the skin or at mucosal sites. This process is generally reversible within a few hours and is not accompanied by tissue destruction. In some cases, the immediate reaction is followed by a so-called late phase reaction occurring approximately 4–24 hours later. The late-phase reaction is characterized by tissue infiltration with inflammatory cells such as neutrophil, eosinophil and basophil granulocytes and mononuclear cells. It is believed that, in particular, the late-phase component of allergic reactions is responsible for tissue destruction, organ dysfunction and persisting clinical symptoms. The phases of allergic reactions have been studied extensively in human skin and respiratory mucosa (Metzger et al, 1985; Charlesworth et al, 1989). It is likely that similar mechanisms occur at the intestinal mucosa, which has been rarely examined in this respect (Crowe and Perdue, 1992).

Figure 1 summarizes the current concept of pathogenesis of allergic reactions. The mechanism of sensitization is still poorly understood. On the basis of in vitro studies we can define several factors which positively (IL-4 and the cell-surface molecule CD40 expressed by TH2-type lymphocytes, mast cells and basophils) and negatively (interferon γ derived from TH1-type lymphocytes and IL-12 from NK-cells) regulate IgE synthesis in B lymphocytes (Romagnani, 1990; Gauchat et al, 1993). More recent studies indicate that neurohormones such as ACTH are also involved in the regulation of human IgE synthesis. The immediate phase of allergic reactions is dependent on mast cell activation through the high-affinity IgE receptor. Apart from IgE-dependent activation, other triggers for human mucosal mast cells could not be identified. However, very recently, we and others found that stem cell factor, also termed *c-kit* ligand, is a potent regulator of human lung and intestinal mast cell function. Stem cell factor

I. Sensitization phase

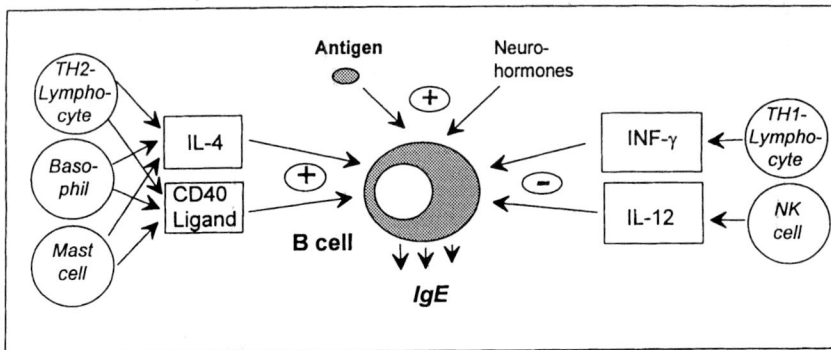

II. Effector phase of allergic reaction

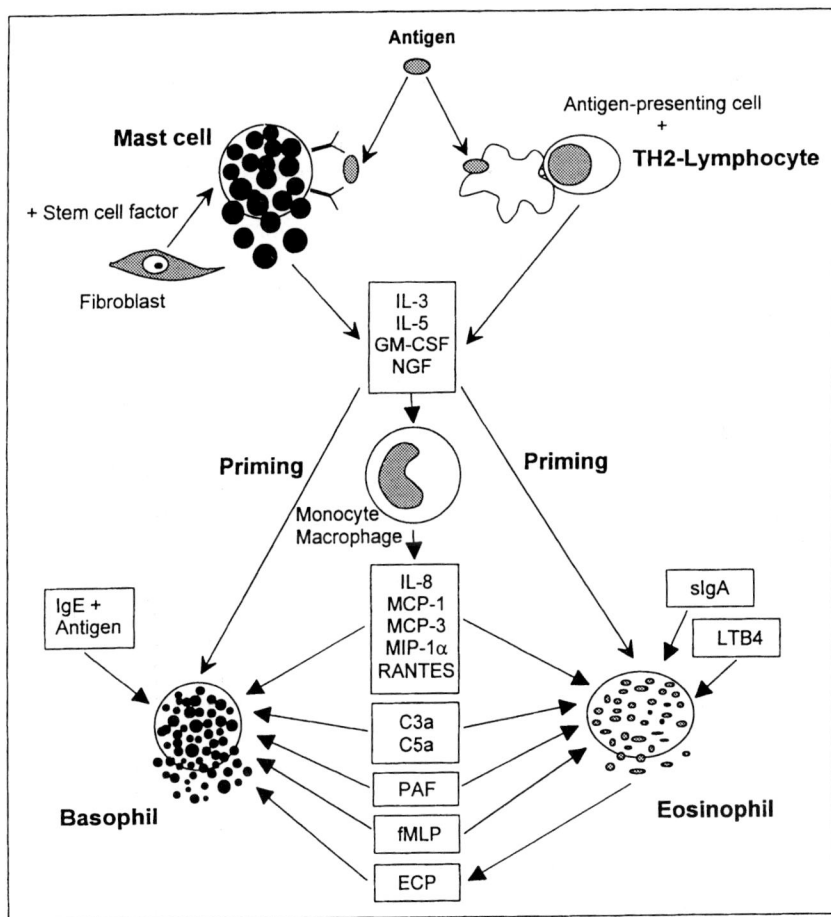

Figure 1. Phases of the allergic reaction (for explanation see text).

potentiates the IgE-dependent mediator release, and, under particular conditions, it induces histamine release also by itself (Bischoff and Dahinden, 1992a,b; Bischoff et al, 1996a). The clinically most relevant late-phase reaction involves not only mast cells, but also allergen-reactive TH2 lymphocytes producing cytokines (IL-3, IL-5, GM-CSF), monocytes, which are the major source of chemokines (IL-8; monocyte-chemotactic protein 1 and 3, MCP-1 and MCP-3; macrophage-inflammatory peptide 1α, MIP-1α; and RANTES), and granulocytes. In particular, eosinophil and basophil granulocytes accumulate at sites of allergic inflammation; they are primed for enhanced mediator release by cytokines (IL-3, IL-5, GM-CSF and nerve growth factor, NGF) and triggered by allergen, chemokines and other humoral factors for the release of inflammatory mediators inducing tissue destruction and organ dysfunction (Bischoff et al, 1990a,b; Takafuji et al, 1991; Rot et al, 1992; Bischoff et al 1993, 1996a). Allergic inflammation is morphologically characterized by the accumulation and activation of eosinophils, basophils and mast cells, but finally involves multiple immunocompetent and inflammatory cells, a complex cellular interaction which is becoming understood more and more.

BIOLOGY OF HUMAN MAST CELLS AND EOSINOPHILS

Several recent in vitro studies have enhanced our understanding of the biology of human mucosal mast cells and eosinophils. Eosinophils can be divided into normodense (resting) eosinophils and hypodense eosinophils, the latter of which are thought to be activated by cytokines or other stimuli (Fukuda and Gleich, 1989). The heterogeneity of mast cells is more complicated (Befus et al, 1985; Irani et al, 1989). At least two major forms of human mast cell exist; they can be distinguished by their protease content. Mast cells containing tryptase and chymase are found mainly in the skin and intestinal submucosa (also termed 'connective-tissue-type mast cells'), whereas mast cells containing tryptase only represent 90% of lung mast cells and almost all mast cells of the intestinal mucosa ('mucosal mast cells'). A third small population was described in intestinal mucosa, which contains chymase, but no tryptase (Bischoff et al, 1996b). Although mast cells are also heterogeneous in terms of functional properties, morphological and functional classifications of human mast cells do not match exactly. However, for skin mast cells several IgE-independent triggering agents, such as C5a or substance P, have been described, which are ineffective in lung and intestinal mast cells (Schulman et al, 1988; Bischoff et al, 1996a). The present overview is focused on mucosal mast cells of intestinal (and lung) tissue, and therefore skin mast cells will not be described further. The development of the human mucosal mast cell from bone-marrow-derived progenitors is not fully understood. Studies, derived mostly from animal models, showed that stem cell factor and IL-3 are important regulators of mast cell proliferation and differentiation (Galli, 1993). In addition, other cytokines such as nerve growth factor may be involved (Matsuda et al, 1991). In contrast to murine mast cells, mature human mast cells lack the IL-3 receptor (Valent et al, 1990). The only cytokine known to regulate mature human mast cell function is stem cell factor, which is capable of inducing mediator release and chemotaxis and which potentiates IgE-receptor-mediated effects (Bischoff and Dahinden, 1992a,b; Bischoff et al, 1996a). Mast cells are tissue cells, and they exert their biological effects by releasing preformed and de novo synthesized mediators upon stimulation. Figure 2 summarizes the most important mast cell-derived mediators such as histamine, proteases, proteoglycans and metabolites of the arachidonic acid cascade known to have potent pro-inflammatory effects (Harvima and Schwartz, 1993). Of particular importance is the recent finding that mast cells, besides their pro-inflammatory

Agonists: Mediators:

Agonists	Mediators
Stem cell factor (*c-kit* ligand)	Histamine Tryptase, Chymase Carboxypeptidase Cathepsin G-like protein Heparin Chondroitin sulphate A+E *(Leukotrienes D4/E4/B4)* Tumour necrosis factor α (TNF α) *Interleukin 4 and 13 (IL-4, IL-13)*

Mast cell

	Leukotriene C4 (LTC4) *Prostaglandin D2 (PGD2)* *Interleukin 3 (IL-3)** *Interleukin 5 (IL-5)** *GM-CSF**
IgE - crosslinking by antigen	

Eosinophil

	Oxygen free radicals Eosinophil peroxidase (EPO) Eosinophil cationic protein (ECP) Eosinophil protein X (EPX) Major basic protein (MBP) *Prostaglandin E2 (PGE2)* *Thromboxane A2 (TxA2)* *Platelet-activating factor (PAF)* *Transforming growth factor (TGF α/b)*
s IgA C3a, C5a fMLP PAF, LTB4 Chemokines IL-3, IL-5 GM-CSF	

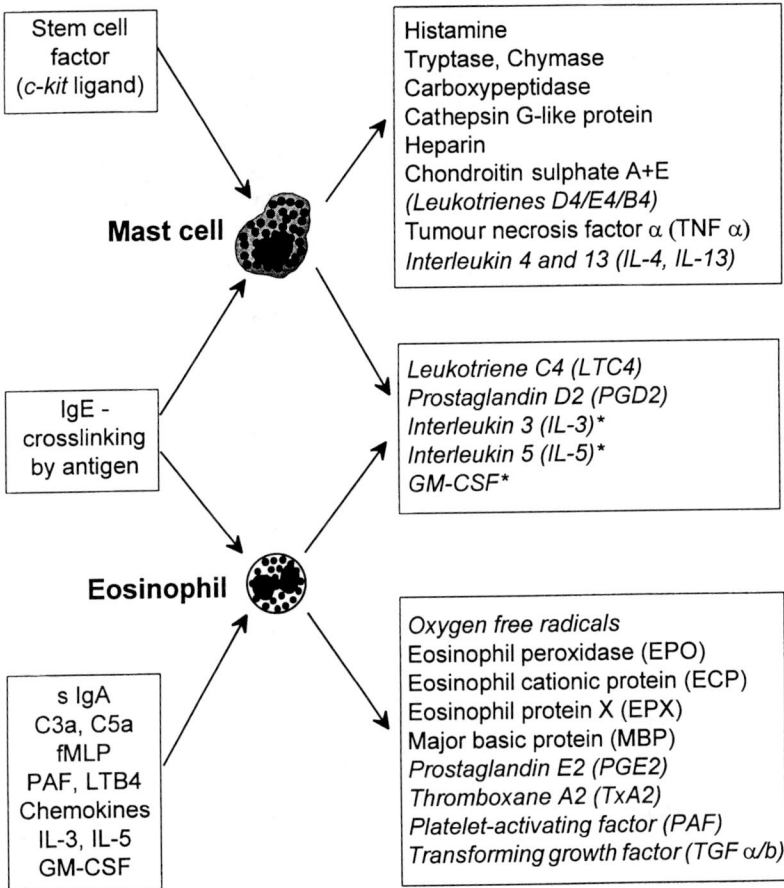

Figure 2. Agonists and mediators of human mucosal mast cells and eosinophil granulocytes. * = in murine mast cells and human eosinophils; de novo-synthesized mediators are printed in italics.

effects, have an immunoregulatory potential by expressing and/or releasing cytokines such as IL-4, IL-13 and CD40 ligand known to be crucial for the regulation of B lymphocytes and induction of IgE synthesis (Brunner et al; 1993; Gauchat et al, 1993; Burd et al, 1995).

Similar observations were made for eosinophils, which, upon appropriate activation, promote inflammation by releasing mediators, for example, cationic proteins, leukotrienes, prostaglandins and platelet-activating factor (PAF), and exerting cytotoxic effects by producing oxygen free-radicals and peroxidase (Weller, 1991). In contrast to mast cells, eosinophils can be activated by multiple immunological and non-immunological agonists, the most important of them being listed in Figure 2 (Abu-Ghazaleh et al, 1989; Takafuji et al, 1991; Rot et al, 1992). On the other hand, eosinophils are a source of multiple cytokines, including TGF α and β, GM-CSF, IL-3 and IL-5 (Weller, 1991). Thus, eosinophils are not only regulated by a particular set of cytokines, but also produce them, partly in an autocrine manner, illustrating a bi-directional link between the specific immune system and inflammatory effector cells. Eosinophils derive from myeloic progenitors, from which they proliferate and differentiate under the influence of IL-5 and, albeit less specifically, IL-3 and GM-CSF (Sanderson, 1993). In contrast to mast cells, they leave the bone marrow as mature cells and remain largely in circulation. Only a few tissues, such as the intestinal mucosa (but not the skin or the respiratory mucosa), contain eosinophils constitutively, the biological function of which is not clear.

PATHOPHYSIOLOGICAL ROLE OF HUMAN MAST CELLS AND EOSINOPHILS

Mast cells and eosinophils are found at multiple body sites, including the GI tract. In contrast, basophils are almost absent in the intestinal mucosa, and therefore they will not be discussed further in this review. The pathophysiological functions of human mast cells and eosinophils, apart from their role in allergic reaction, are largely unclear. It has been suggested that mast cells are involved in tissue repair processes because they accumulate at sites of tissue injuries, wound healing and bone fractures (Severson, 1969). However, it is unknown whether mast cells also promote wound healing in lung or intestinal tissue. In an animal model, histamine supported the restitution of damaged intestinal mucosa (Fujimoto et al, 1992), possibly through suppression of pro-inflammatory cytokines such as TNF α (Vannier et al, 1991). Interestingly, in patients with active ulcerative colitis, an increase in mast cell numbers was found at the line of demarcation between actively inflamed and normal intestinal mucosa (King et al, 1992), further supporting the hypothesis that mast cells promote tissue repair. Mast cell accumulation was also found in fibrotic tissues such as neurofibroma, liver fibrosis, and radiologically induced lung fibromatosis, suggesting a role for mast cells in the induction of fibrotic tissue transformation (Claman, 1985). Furthermore, large numbers of mast cells are found at sites of polyneuropathies (Knorr-Held and Meier, 1990), and

Bienenstock and co-workers have shown that intestinal mast cells are in close anatomical relationship to nerve cells (Williams et al, 1995). It is not yet clear which functional role mast cells play in the 'neuro-immune connection', but the observations clearly indicate that the function of mast cells is not restricted to allergic reactions and pro-inflammatory effects. It is tempting to speculate that mast cells are involved in a number of 'tissue-transforming processes' such as wound healing and fibrosis, the mechanisms of which have yet to be elucidated.

A major biological function of eosinophils is their role in defence against helminths and other parasites, which occur mainly in the GI tract (Butterworth and Thorne, 1993; Liu et al, 1995). The cytotoxic potential of eosinophils enables this type of cell to kill worms such as schistosoma and enterobius vermicularis, the infection of which is characterized by a marked eosinophil accumulation and activation. Interestingly, helminth infections also are often characterized by the induction of IgE synthesis and mast cell accumulation, suggesting some parallels in the pathogenesis of parasitosis and allergy (Ishisaka, 1988). The clinical relevance of parasitic infections, particularly in the Third-world countries, which often start in the intestinal tract, may account for the fact that eosinophils are constitutively present at the intestinal barrier. Allergic reactions are rarely observed in Third-world countries, raising the idea that, in patients from industrial countries, in which parasite infections hardly ever occur, eosinophils develop aberrant reactions to other than parasitic antigens, and thereby prepare the way for acquiring allergic disease (Butterworth and Thorne, 1993). Apart from their role in parasitic infection, eosinophils have been associated with pathologies such as vasculitis and autoimmune disease, and, as in the case of mast cells, with tissue fibrosis (Hall and Walport, 1993).

The role of intestinal eosinophils and mast cells in inflammatory bowel disease is largely unclear. However, mediators derived from eoinophils and mast cells were found to be elevated in intestinal lavage fluids of patients with active Crohn's disease (Hällgren et al, 1989; Fox et al, 1990; Knutson et al, 1990), and an increased luminal release of sulphidoleukotrienes has been reported in patients with inactive Crohn's disease (Casellas et al, 1994). Moreover, a number of morphological studies provide evidence for eosinophil and mast cell activation in Crohn's disease, ulcerative colitis, celiac disease and eosinophilic gastroenteritis (Talley et al, 1992; Dubucquoi et al, 1995; Bischoff et al, 1996b), suggesting that eosinophils and mast cells may be involved in the pathogenesis of at least some forms of inflammatory bowel diseases. In this respect it is interesting to note that, in a histological study performed several years ago, it was suggested that the number of eosinophils in the rectal mucosa predicts the clinical course of ulcerative proctocolitis (Heatley and James, 1978). In addition, other GI pathologies involving accumulation and activation of intestinal eosinophils and/or mast cells have been reported—such as mastocytosis (Cherner et al, 1988), secretory diarrhoea (Clouse et al, 1992; Crowe and Perdue, 1993; Stack et al, 1995), and GI affections induced by chronic alcoholism (Colombel et al, 1988). The diseases in which mast cells and eosinophils are thought to play a role are summarized in Figure 3.

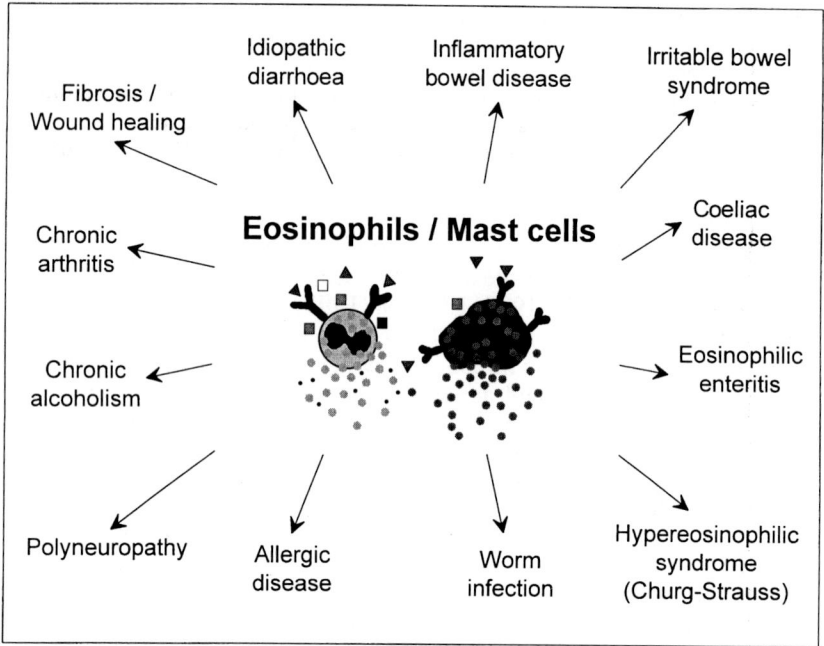

Figure 3. Diseases associated with mast cell and/or eosinophil activation (for references, see text).

DEFINITION, EPIDEMIOLOGY AND DIAGNOSIS OF INTESTINAL ALLERGY

Intestinal allergy is defined as an immunologically mediated adverse reaction to a foreign antigen. If the antigen is food protein, the term '(intestinal) food allergy' is used. Food allergy may be mediated by IgE-dependent mechanisms ('type I hypersensitivity reaction' according to the classification by Coombs and Gell), but other mechanisms such as immune complexes ('type III reactions') or cellular reactions ('type IV reactions') may be involved (Halpern and Scott, 1987; Sampson et al, 1989). According to the recommendations of the European and American Academies of Allergy and Clinical Immunology, other forms of adverse reactions to food-based on non-immunological mechanisms such as pseudoallergic reactions, lactose intolerance or deficiency of glucose-6-phosphate dehydrogenase (6-GPD) should be separated and termed 'food intolerance' (Anderson and Sogn, 1984; Bruijnzeel-Koomen et al, 1995).

The prevalence of food allergy and other forms of intestinal allergy is largely unknown. It has been estimated that, depending on the methods used for diagnosis, 2–5% of the general population suffer from food allergy or food-intolerance reactions (Crowe and Perdue, 1992; Shanahan, 1993). A recent population study of food intolerance in adults reported a prevalence of 1.4% based on a questionnaire involving 20 000 individuals and oral food challenge tests. Of individuals testing positive in the food-challenge test, 28% had intestinal symptoms (Young et al, 1994). However, it has to be considered that 20–45% of the adult population believe that they suffer from adverse reactions to food (Crowe and Perdue, 1992; Shanahan, 1993), indicating the necessity of objective diagnostic means.

The methods available for confirming the diagnosis of gastrointestinal food allergy are at present insufficient, and therefore it remains difficult to identify afflicted patients on an objective basis (Goldman et al, 1987). Since the symptoms of intestinal food allergy are unspecific and variable, the diagnosis is to a large part an 'exclusion diagnosis'. Non-immunological causes of adverse reactions to food have to be excluded by different means, such as the lactose-tolerance test, malabsorption tests, microbiological examinations, sonography and endoscopy. It is well known that the classical allergological means, such as skin tests and measurement of total or specific IgE in serum, are of limited value for confirming the diagnosis of food allergy. Elevated total IgE or high levels of specific IgE may argue for the presence of intestinal food allergy. However, normal values of such parameters or negative skin tests do not exclude intestinal food allergy, as shown by several studies (Goldman et al, 1987; Sampson, 1988; Bock, 1995). In 375 patients with gastrointestinal disease (Crohn's disease, ulcerative colitis, and other intestinal disease of unknown aetiology) we found that most had almost normal total serum IgE concentrations and rather low levels, if any, of specific IgE (own unpublished observation). Eosinophilia in peripheral blood or intestinal tissue may suggest an allergic aetiology, but is not specific (Crowe and Perdue, 1992). A probationary treatment with disodium cromoglycate (DSCG, oral dose 4×200 mg) may also be used as a diagnostic means, since DSCG is believed to improve specifically allergic symptoms.

Oral challenge tests with food substances are acknowledged as the 'gold standard' for the confirmation of food allergy (Sampson, 1988; Bock, 1995). However, these tests are often not pragmatic in practice, they are time-consuming and expensive, and involve the risk of anaphylaxis. Even more importantly, their read-out system depends on the patients' subjective symptoms, and therefore, despite the fact that such tests can be performed in a double-blind placebo-controlled fashion, they remain subjective. The only objective method for confirming a diagnosis of adverse reaction to food is by elimination diet and re-challenge. In practice, however, this approach has limitations because of difficulties in eliminating the food allergen(s) suspected to be of relevance, which depends on a correct choice of the food to be avoided, the compliance of the patient, and the type of food. To avoid fatal reactions, patients have to be carefully selected, and challenges should be performed in hospital settings (David, 1984).

Several attempts have been made to improve the diagnosis of intestinal food allergy by establishing new laboratory methods such as measurement of IgE or eosinophil-derived mediators in stool samples (Kolmannskog and Haneberg, 1985; Berstad et al, 1993; André et al, 1995), determination of specific IgG and IgA against food antigens in serum (Knoflach et al, 1987), analysis of in vitro mediator release by peripheral blood basophils or intestinal mast cells upon challenge with food antigens (Selbekk, 1985; Nolte et al, 1989; Baenkler and Lux, 1989), or assessment of intestinal permeability (André et al, 1987). Most of these tests are either very complicated to perform, or their validity has not been confirmed yet by clinical studies, but some of the tests provided new insights into the mechanisms of intestinal allergy or may be useful for future clinical studies.

To improve the diagnostic means for confirming intestinal food allergy, we developed a new diagnostic approach, the colonoscopic allergen provocation test (COLAP test). Provocation tests are established for the nasal, conjunctival and bronchial mucosa, and their value for confirming the diagnosis of allergic disease and for identifying allergens of relevance is well recognized. A few attempts have been made to develop similar tests for the gastrointestinal mucosa, but they could not be established for clinical practice (Pollard and Stuart, 1942; Reimann et al, 1985; Romanski, 1987; Bagnato et al, 1995). In the COLAP test, the caecal mucosa is challenged endoscopically with three food antigen extracts, a buffer control and a positive control (histamine). The mucosal weal and flare reaction is registered semiquantitatively 20 minutes after challenge. We performed the COLAP test in 45 adult patients with abdominal symptoms suspected of being related to food allergy, and in five healthy volunteers. No systemic anaphylactic reactions were observed in response to intestinal challenge. The COLAP test was positive to at least one food antigen in 35 out of 45 patients (78%), whereas no reaction in response to antigen was observed in healthy volunteers. Antigen-induced weal-and-flare reactions were correlated with intestinal mast cell and eosinophil activation, and with patients' history of adverse reactions to food, but not with serum levels of total or specific IgE or skin-test results. The data suggest that the COLAP test may be a useful diagnostic procedure in patients with suspected intestinal food allergy and a new tool for the study of underlying mechanisms (Bischoff et al, manuscript submitted for publication).

Despite the limitations of almost all diagnostic means discussed here, most of them should be performed because each may provide some information, and only the synopsis of all findings allows the final diagnosis. On the basis of our present knowledge, we propose a flow diagram used successfully in our department for the diagnosis of intestinal food allergy (Figure 4).

CLINICAL IMPLICATIONS FOR THE GASTROINTESTINAL TRACT

The clinical manifestation of intestinal food allergy is variable; the symptoms are rather non-specific, and they include abdominal pain, cramps, flatulence, irregular bowel movements, intestinal blood loss and malabsorption syndrome. According to our own experience, the most relevant allergens for intestinal food allergy are milk proteins, hazelnut, wheat, apple, pork and egg. Apart from the GI tract, other organ systems such as the skin, the respiratory mucosa, and possibly also the central

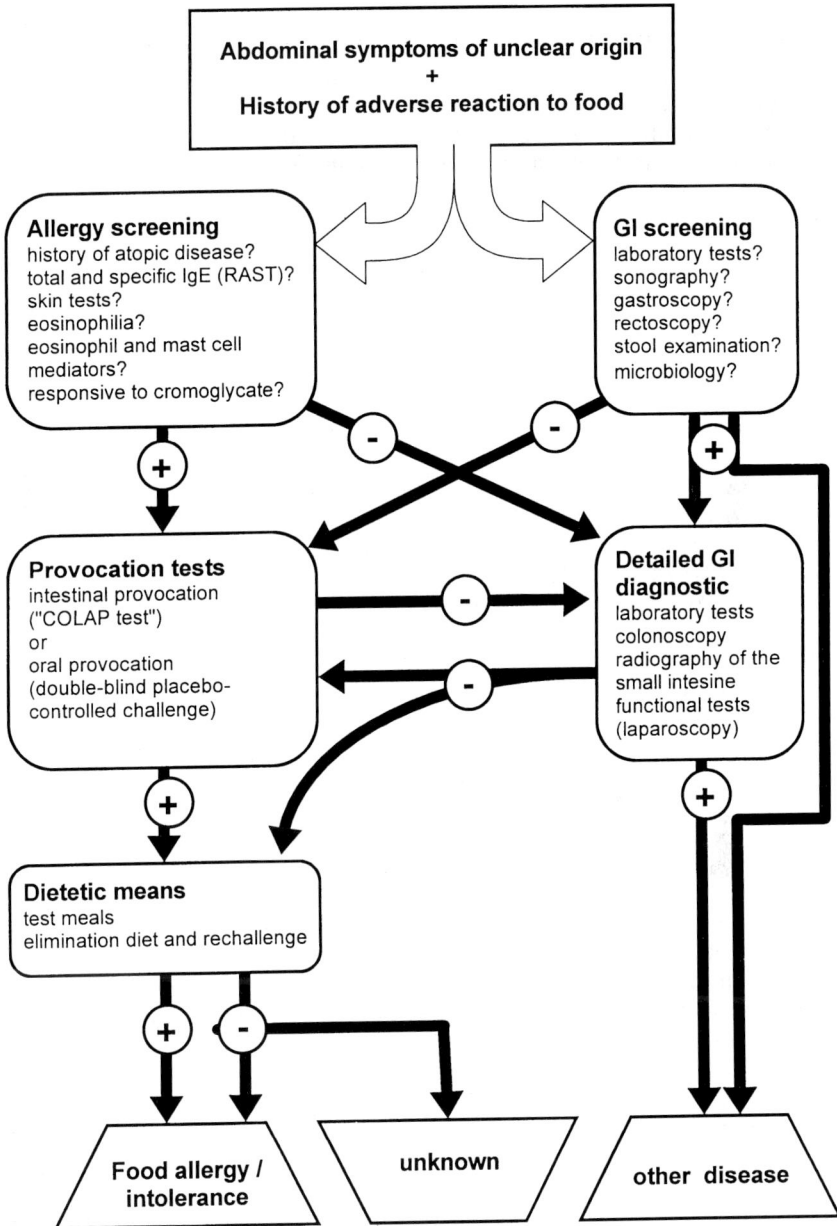

Figure 4. Flow diagram for the diagnosis of intestinal food allergy (further explanation in the text).

nervous system may be involved (Crowe and Perdue, 1992). Allergic diseases manifestating primarily outside the GI tract may also affect the intestinal mucosa. For example, patients with bronchial asthma have duodenal pathological abnormalities similar to those observed in the bronchial mucosa, suggesting that the whole mucosal immune system is involved in allergic disease (Wallaert et al, 1995). Similar observations have been made in Crohn's disease, which is frequently accompanied by a latent pulmonary involvement (Bonniere et al, 1986). In practice, several GI diseases, which have been listed in Figure 5, have to be considered (and excluded) in the differential diagnosis of intestinal (food) allergy.

Differential diagnosis of intestinal allergy

Food allergy: Pseudoallergic reactions to food
                          Toxic reactions (e.g. bacterial contamination of food)
                          Enzyme deficiencies (e.g. lactase or 6-GDP deficiency)

Other intestinal   Crohn's disease
hypersensitivity   Ulcerative colitis
reactions: Celiac disease
                          Eosinophilic gastroenteritis
                          Irritable bowel syndrome
                          Infectious gastroenteritis
                          Collagenous colitis
                          Porphyria
                          Dumping syndrome

Figure 5. Differential diagnosis of intestinal allergy.

The mechanisms underlying intestinal food allergy are largely unclear, although it may be anticipated that similar mechanisms are involved as described for other forms of allergic disease. However, they may be different to classical type I hypersensitivity reactions of the skin or the respiratory mucosa, since many patients with evidence of food allergy have negative skin tests, and rather low IgE levels in serum. To explain this observation it is possible to envisage two hypotheses which are not mutually exclusive: either specific IgE is present only in the intestinal mucosa but not systemically (Kolmannskog and Haneberg, 1985), or intestinal reactions are not (or not only) mediated by an IgE-dependent mechanism (Halpern and Scott, 1987).

The role of IgE in GI allergy is unclear at present, but several studies clearly indicated that eosinophils and mast cells are involved. Therefore, measurement of eosinophil and mast cell mediators may be more appropriate than IgE measurements for the diagnosis and monitoring of intestinal allergic diseases. There is ample evidence that eosinophil and mast cell activation occurs not only in allergic disease, but also in a number of other GI pathologies. It is evident that such findings do not yet indicate that allergic mechanisms are involved; however, allergic diseases should be considered in the differential diagnosis of GI symptoms of unclear origin. In conclusion, intestinal mast cell and eosinophil activation seems to be an important event in the pathophysiology of different GI diseases, which requires further investigation.

SUMMARY

Despite the progress made in understanding the mechanisms of allergic disease, the pathophysiology and clinical significance of intestinal allergic reactions is largely unclear. The intestinal mucosa is pre-destined for allergic reactions against food proteins and other antigens, and a number of studies indicate that allergic reactions occur in the GI tract. However, only a few epidemiological data are available, and the mechanisms are poorly understood. Intestinal allergic reactions may be different to classical IgE-mediated reactions because patients with intestinal allergy often have negative skin tests and low levels of serum IgE. There is increasing evidence that, as with the findings in the skin and lung, mast cells and eosinophils play a central role in mediating intestinal allergic reactions. Furthermore, both types of cell are found to be activated in a number of other GI inflammatory diseases such as inflammatory bowel disease, celiac disease and eosinophilic gastroenteritis. However, the relationship between these pathologies and intestinal allergy is largely unclear. A major clinical problem is the lack of appropriate means for confirming the diagnosis of intestinal allergy. However, new test systems have been developed—such as the measurement of eosinophil mediators in stool samples or endoscopic provocation tests performed locally at the intestinal mucosa, which may improve the possibility of identifying afflicted patients on an objective basis. Since symptoms of intestinal allergic reactions are variable and non-specific, the diagnosis requires the use of multiple tests and the exclusion of other pathologies such as infectious disease or non-immunological intolerance reactions. The preferred therapeutic option is avoidance of the allergens of relevance; however, this approach can be realized only in some patients, whereas others require additional treatment, for example, with oral cromoglycate or corticosteroids. Although we do not yet know to what extent intestinal allergic reactions may be an aetiological factor in GI diseases, such reactions should be considered in the differential diagnosis of unclear intestinal inflammation and irritable bowel syndrome.

Acknowledgement

We thank J. Mayer, A. Herrmann, J. Wedemeyer, A. Bendjah, M. Hoffman, J. Grabowsky and K. Rifai for their contribution, G. Weier and K. Wordelmann for their expert technical assistance, and P. N. Meier, M. Gebel and the endoscopy unit for their excellent co-operation. The work was supported in part by the Deutsche Forschungsgemeinschaft, Bonn, Germany (grant SFB280-C8 to S.C.B.) and by the Else-Kröner-Stiftung, Bad Homburg, Germany (grant to S.C.B. and M.P.M.).

REFERENCES

Abu-Ghazaleh RI, Fujisawa T, Mestecky J et al (1989) IgA-induced eosinophil degranulation. *Journal of Immunology* **142:** 2393–2400.

Anderson JA & Sogn DD (1984) Adverse reactions to foods. *American Academy of Allergy and Immunology Commitee on Adverse Reactions to Foods. Bethesda, MD, National Institute of Allergy and Infectious Diseases, National Institute of Health,* NIH Publication No. 84-2442.

André C, André F, Colin L & Cavagna S (1987) Measurement of intestinal permeability to mannitol and lactulose as a means of diagnosing food allergy and evaluating therapeutic effectiveness of disodium cromoglycate. *Annals of Allergy* **59:** 127–130.

André F, André C & Cavagna S (1995) IgE in stools as indicator of food sensitization. *Allergy* **50:** 328–333.

Baenkler HW & Lux G (1989) Antigen-induced histamine release from duodenal biopsy in gastrointestinal food allergy. *Annals of Allergy* **62:** 449–452.

Bagnato GF, Di Cesare E, Caruso RA et al (1995) Gastric mucosal mast cells in atopic subjects. *Allergy* **50:** 322–327.

Befus D, Goodacre R, Dyck N & Bienenstock J (1985) Mast cell heterogeneity in man. *International Archives of Allergy and Applied Immunology* **76:** 232–236.

Berstad A, Borkje B, Riedel B et al (1993) Increased fecal eosinophil cationic protein in inflammatory bowel disease. *Hepato-Gastroenterology* **40:** 276–278.

Bischoff SC & Dahinden CA (1992a) C-kit ligand: a unique potentiator of mediator release by human lung mast cells. *Journal of Experimental Medicine* **175:** 237–244.

Bischoff SC & Dahinden CA (1992b) Effect of c-kit ligand on mediator release by human lung mast cells. *International Archives of Allergy and Immunology* **99:** 319–322.

Bischoff SC, De Weck AL & Dahinden CA (1990a) Interleukin 3 and granulocyte/macrophage-colony-stimulating factor render human basophils responsive to low concentrations of complement component C3a. *Proceedings of the National Academy of Science of the USA.* **87:** 6813–6817.

Bischoff SC, Brunner T, De Weck AL & Dahinden CA (1990b) Interleukin 5 modifies histamine release and leukotriene generation by human basophils in response to diverse agonists. *Journal of Experimental Medicine* **172:** 1577–1582.

Bischoff SC, Krieger M, Brunner T et al (1993) RANTES and related chemokines activate human basophil granulocytes through different G protein-coupled receptors. *European Journal of Immunology* **23:** 761–767.

Bischoff SC, Schwengberg S, Wordelmann K et al (1996a). Effect of c-kit ligand, stem cell factor, on mediator release by human intestinal mast cells isolated from patients with inflammatory bowel disease and controls. *Gut* **38:** 104–114.

Bischoff SC, Wedemeyer J, Herrmann A et al (1996b) Quantitative assessment of intestinal eosinophils and mast cells in inflammatory bowel disease. *Histopathology* **28:** 1–13.

Bock SA (1995) Food challenges in the diagnosis of food hypersensitivity. In De Weck AL & Sampson HA (eds) *Intestinal Immunology and Food Allergy,* pp 105–117. New York: Raven Press.

Bonniere P, Wallaert B, Cortot A et al (1986) Latent pulmonary involvement in Crohn's disease: biological, functional, bronchoalveolar lavage and scintigraphic studies. *Gut* **27:** 919–925.

Brandtzaeg P, Halstensen TS, Kett K et al (1989) Immunobiology and immunopathology of human gut mucosa: humoral immunity and intraepthelial lymphocytes. *Gastroenterology* **97:** 1562–1584.

Bruijnzeel-Koomen C, Ortolani C, Aas K et al (1995) Adverse reactions to food. *Allergy* **50:** 623–635.

Brunner T, Heusser CH & Dahinden CA (1993) Human peripheral blood basophils primed by IL-3 produce IL-4 in response to immunoglobulin E receptor stimulation. *Journal of Experimental Medicine* **177:** 605–611.

Burd PR, Thompson WC, Max EE & Mills FC (1995) Activated mast cells produce interleukin 13. *Journal of Experimental Medicine* **181:** 1373–1380.

Butterworth AE & Thorne KJI (1993) Eosinophils and parasitic diseases. In Smith H & Cook RM (eds) *Immunopharmacology of Eosinophils,* pp 119–150. London: Academic Press.

Casellas F, Guarner F, Antolin M et al (1994) Abnormal leukotriene C4 release by unaffected jejunal mucosa in patients with inactive Crohn's disease. *Gut* **35:** 517–522.

Charlesworth EN, Hood AF, Soter NA et al (1989) Cutaneous late-phase response to allergen.

Mediator release and inflammatory cell infiltration. *Journal of Clinical Investigation* **83:** 1519–1526.

Cherner JA, Jensen RT, Dubois A et al (1988) Gastrointestinal dysfunction in systemic mastocytosis. A prospective study. *Gastroenterology* **95:** 657–667.

Claman HN (1985) Mast cells, T cells and abnormal fibrosis. *Immunology Today* **6:** 192–195.

Clouse RE, Alpers DH, Hockenbery DM et al (1992) Pericrypt eosinophilic enterocolitis and chronic diarrhea. *Gastroenterology* **103:** 168–176.

Colombel JF, Hällgren R, Venge P et al (1988) Neutrophil and eosinophil involvement of the small bowel affected by chronic alcoholism. *Gut* **29:** 1656–1660.

Crowe SE & Perdue MH (1992) Gastrointestinal food hypersensitivity: basic mechanisms of pathophysiology. *Gastroenterology* **103:** 1075–1095.

Crowe SE & Perdue MH (1993) Anti-immunoglobulin E-stimulated ion transport in human large and small intestine. *Gastroenterology* **105:** 764–772.

David TJ (1984) Anaphylactic shock during elimination diets for severe atopic dermatitis. *Archives of Diseases in Children* **59:** 983–986.

Dubucquoi S, Janin A, Klein O et al (1995) Activated eosinophils and interleukin 5 expression in early recurrence of Crohn's disease. *Gut* **37:** 242–246.

Fantry GT & James SP (1994) Cell-mediated immunity and mucosal immunity. *Current Opinion in Gastroenterology* **10:** 365–373.

Farah DA, Calder I, Benson L & Mackenzie JF (1985) Specific food intolerances: its place as a cause of gastrointestinal symptoms. *Gut* **26:** 164–168.

Ferguson A (1990) Food sensitivity or self-deception? *New England Journal of Medicine* **323:** 476–478.

Fox CC, Lazenby AJ, Moore WC et al (1990) Enhancement of human intestinal mast cell mediator release in active ulcerative colitis. *Gastroenterology* **99:** 119–124.

Fujimoto K, Imamura I, Granger DN et al (1992) Histamine and histidine decarboxylase are correlated with mucosal repair in rat small intestine after ischemia-reperfusion. *Journal of Clinical Investigation* **89:** 126–133.

Fukuda T & Gleich GJ (1989) Heterogeneity of human eosinophils. *Journal of Allergy and Clinical Immunology* **83:** 369–373.

Galli SJ (1993) New concepts about the mast cell. *New England Journal of Medicine* **328:** 257–265.

Gauchat JF, Henchoz S, Mazzei G et al (1993) Induction of human IgE synthesis in B cells by mast cells and basophils. *Nature* **365:** 340–343.

Goldman AS, Kantal AG, Ham Pong AJ & Goldblum RM (1987) Food hypersensitivities: historical perspectives, diagnosis and clinical presentation. In Brostoff J & Challacombe SJ (eds) *Food Allergy and Intolerance*, pp 797–805. London: W. B. Saunders.

Hall FC & Walport MJ (1993) Hypereosinophilic syndromes: association with vasculitis, fibrosis and autoimmunity. *Clinical and Experimental Allergy* **23:** 542–547.

Hällgren R, Colombel JF, Dahl R et al (1989) Neutrophil and eosinophil involvement of the small bowel in patients with celiac disease and Crohn's disease: studies on the secretion rate and immunhistochemical localization of granulocyte granule constituents. *American Journal of Medicine* **86:** 56–64.

Halpern GM & Scott JR (1987) Non-IgE antibody mediated mechanisms in food allergy. *Annals of Allergy* **58:** 14–27.

Harvima RJ & Schwartz LB (1993) Mast cell-derived mediators. In Foreman J (ed.) *Immunopharmacology of Mast Cells and Basophils*, pp 115–138. London: Academic Press.

Heatley RV & James PD (1978) Eosinophils in the rectal mucosa. A simple method of predicting the outcome of ulcerative proctocolitis? *Gut* **20:** 787–791.

Irani AA, Bradford TR, Kepley CL et al (1989) Detection of MC_T and MC_{TC} types of human mast cells by immunohistochemistry using new monoclonal anti-tryptase and anti-chymase antibodies. *Journal of Histochemistry and Cytochemistry* **37:** 1509–1515.

Ishisaka K (1988) IgE-binding factors and regulation of the IgE antibody response. *Annual Reviews in Immunology* **6:** 513–534.

King T, Biddle W, Bhatia P et al (1992) Colonic mucosal mast cell distribution at line demarcation of active ulcerative colitis. *Digestive Diseases and Science* **37:** 490–495.

Knoflach P, Park BH, Cunningham R et al (1987) Serum antibodies to cow's milk proteins in ulcerative colitis and Crohn's disease. *Gastroenterology* **92:** 479–485.

Knorr-Held S & Meier C (1990) Mast cells in human polyneuropathies: their density and regional distribution. *Clinical Neuropathology* **9:** 121–124.

Knutson L, Ahrenstedt Ö, Odling B & Hällgren R (1990) The jejunal secretion of histamine is increased in active Crohn's disease. *Gastroenterology* **98:** 849–854.

Kolmannskog S & Haneberg B (1985) Immunoglobulin E in faeces from children with allergy. Evidence of local production of IgE in the gut. *International Archives of Allergy and Applied Immunology* **76:** 133–137.

Liu LX, Chi J, Upton MP & Ash LR (1995) Eosinophilic colitis associated with larvae of the pinworm enterobius vermicularis. *Lancet* **346:** 410–412.

Matsuda H, Kannan Y, Ushio H et al (1991) Nerve growth factor induces development of connective tissue-type mast cells in vitro from murine bone marrow cells. *Journal of Experimental Medicine* **174:** 7–14.

Metzger WJ, Hunninghake GW & Richerson HB (1985) Late asthmatic responses: inquiry into mechanisms and significance. *Clinical Reviews of Allergy* **3:** 145–165.

Nolte H, Schiotz PO, Kruse A et al (1989) Comparison of intestinal mast cell and basophil histamine release in children with food allergic reactions. *Allergy* **44:** 554–565.

Pollard HM & Stuart GJ (1942) Experimental reproduction of gastric allergy in human beings with controlled observations on the mucosa. *Journal of Allergy* **13:** 467–473.

Reimann HJ, Ring J, Ultsch B & Wendt P (1985) Intragastral provocation under endoscopic control (IPEC) in food allergy: mast cell and histamine changes in gastric mucosa. *Clinical Allergy* **15:** 195–202.

Romagnani S (1990) Regulation and deregulation of human IgE synthesis. *Immunology Today* **11:** 316–321.

Romanski B (1987) The pathology of food allergy studied by gastric allergen challenge. In Brostoff J & Challacombe SJ (eds) *Food Allergy and Intolerance*, pp 917–931. London: W. B. Saunders.

Rot A, Krieger M, Brunner T et al (1992) RANTES und macrophage inflammatory protein 1α induce the migration and activation of normal human eosinophil granulocytes. *Journal of Experimental Medicine* **176:** 1489–1495.

Sampson HA (1988) Immunologically mediated food allergy: the importance of food challenge procedures. *Annals of Allergy* **60:** 262–269.

Sampson HA, Broadbent KR & Bernhisel-Broadbent J (1989) Spontaneous release of histamine from basophils and histamine-releasing factor in patients with atopic dermatitis and food hypersensitivity. *New England Journal of Medicine* **321:** 228–232.

Sampson HA, Mendelson L & Rosen JP (1992) Fatal and near-fatal anaphylactic reactions to food in children and adolescents. *New England Journal of Medicine* **327:** 380–384.

Sanderson CJ (1993) Interleukin-5 and the regulation of eosinophil production. In Smith H & Cook RM (eds) *Immunopharmacology of Eosinophils*, pp 11–24. London: Academic Press.

Schulman ES, Post TJ, Henson PM & Giclas PC (1988) Differential effects of the complement peptides, C5a and C5a des arg on human basophil and lung mast cell histamine release. *Journal of Clinical Investigation* **81:** 918–923.

Selbekk BH (1985) A comparison between in vitro jejunal mast cell degranulation and intragastric challenge in patients with suspected food intolerance. *Scandinavian Journal of Gastroenterology* **20:** 299–303.

Severson AR (1969) Mast cells in areas of experimental bone resorption and remodelling. *British Journal of Experimental Pathology* **50:** 17–21.

Shanahan F (1993) Food allergy: fact, fiction, and fatality. *Gastroenterology* **104:** 1229–1231.

Stack WA, Keely SJ, O'Donoghue DP & Baird AW (1995) Immune regulation of human colonic electrolyte transport in vitro. *Gut* **36:** 395–400.

Takafuji S, Bischoff SC, De Weck AL & Dahinden CA (1991) IL-3 and IL-5 prime normal human eosinophils to produce leukotriene C4 in response to soluble agonists. *Journal of Immunology* **147:** 3855–3861.

Talley NJ, Kephart GM, McGovern TW et al (1992) Deposition of eosinophil granule major basic protein in eosinophilic gastroenteritis and celiac disease. *Gastroenterology* **103:** 137–145.

Valent P, Besemer J, Sillaber C et al (1990) Failure to detect IL-3 binding sites on human mast cells. *Journal of Immunology* **145:** 3432–3437.

Vannier E, Miller LC & Dinarello CA (1991) Histamine supresses gene expression and synthesis of tumor necrosis factor alpha via histamine H2 receptors. *Journal of Experimental Medicine* **174:** 281–284.

Wallaert B, Desreumaux P, Copin MC et al (1995) Immunoreactivity for interleukin 3 and 5 and granulocyte/macrophage colony-stimulating factor of intestinal mucosa in bronchial asthma. *Journal of Experimental Medicine* **182:** 1897–1904.

Weller PF (1991) The immunobiology of eosinophils. *New England Journal of Medicine* **324:** 1110–1118.

Williams RM, Bienenstock J & Stead RH (1995) Mast cells: the neuroimmune connection. In Marone G (ed.) *Human Basophils and Mast Cells: Biological Aspects*, pp 208–235. Basel: Karger.

Young E, Stoneham MD, Petruckevitch A et al (1994) A population study of food intolerance. *Lancet* **343:** 1127–1130.

5

Immunopathology of primary biliary cirrhosis

CLAUDIO GALPERIN
M. ERIC GERSHWIN

Autoimmune diseases are believed to be caused by a failure of the immune system to distinguish between self, for which there exists a state of natural immune tolerance, and non-self. Failure of immune tolerance often results in adverse consequences, including tissue and organ destruction resulting from abnormalities of both humoral and cell-mediated immune responses. Primary biliary cirrhosis (PBC) is the quintessential example of an organ-specific autoimmune disease, a group of disorders in which the antigen is broadly distributed to virtually all nucleated cells, but the immune destruction is specifically targeted to relatively few tissues. The auto-antigens recognized in PBC are predominantly components of normal mitochondria, although less commonly components of the nucleus and cytoplasm are also recognized. How a mitochondrial antigen, physically sheltered from the immune system by two membrane barriers, can elicit an immune response or, once tolerance is broken, how this 'self-reactive' immunity causes tissue damage in only some cells, is still unknown. Undeniably, however, in PBC immune damage is directed almost exclusively to the intrahepatic biliary epithelium.

Recent advances in molecular immunology, together with other emerging technologies (such as affinity mass spectrometry), have been of cardinal importance in elucidating the identity of the autoantigens and the epitopes on the molecules targeted by T and B cell responses in PBC. Nonetheless, the primary event that leads to disease remains unknown. The present difficulties in better understanding the effector mechanisms involved in the pathogenesis of PBC stem, to a large extent, from our inability to examine the disease in its earliest stages and throughout its evolution. When patients first come to the attention of the clinician, the disease is believed to have been present for years to decades. Thus, when we come to dissect the immune response, we are observing the end-stages of a process, and many of the immune responses we can detect may result from 'bystander' or secondary response to cellular components released from dying cells. In this chapter we will focus mainly on a discussion of recent data which have provided a basis for defining the autoimmune response in PBC and information which suggests an explanation for the phenomenon of selective immune damage.

Baillière's Clinical Gastroenterology—
Vol. 10, No. 3, September 1996
ISBN 0–7020–2187–3
0950–3528/96/030461 + 21 $12.00/00

461

CLINICAL ASPECTS

Primary biliary cirrhosis is an autoimmune destructive disease of the intra-hepatic bile ducts characterized by inflammation of the portal triads of the liver followed by fibrosis and, eventually, liver failure. Of remarkable female predominance, PBC is virtually the only autoimmune disease never reported in paediatric patients. Cases under the age of 30 are exceptional, and the incidence progressively rises with age. The onset of disease is often marked by the presence of lethargy and debilitating pruritus, with jaundice eventually occurring as the disease progresses. Liver failure and portal hypertension ultimately develop in most patients with PBC. The manifestations of these disorders are similar to those in other patients with end-stage cirrhosis, although patients with PBC who bleed from oesophageal varices appear to be better candidates for portosystemic anastomosis, and are less likely to develop hepatic encephalopathy (Spinsi et al, 1981; Sepersky et al, 1982). Patients with long-standing disease have additional morbidity due to the high prevalence of steatorrhoea, osteomalacia and osteoporosis. Moreover, PBC patients also have a higher-than-expected frequency of other presumed autoimmune conditions, such as Sjögren's syndrome and scleroderma/CREST syndrome. Further clinical associations include renal tubular acidosis and increased frequency of hepatocellular carcinoma in males. Although most PBC patients fit into the classic clinical picture described herein, the natural history and time course of the disease progression can vary widely among patients. Furthermore, as a result of increased awareness of the disease and widespread use of multiphasic laboratory screening tests, an increasing number of patients have been detected in the pre-symptomatic stage of disease.

DIAGNOSIS

Primary biliary cirrhosis is readily suspected in women who present with persistent pruritus, hepatosplenomegaly and jaundice, and whose bio-chemical liver function tests demonstrate a cholestatic pattern. The serum alkaline phosphatase and gamma-glutamyltranspeptidase values are invariably elevated, often to striking levels. Alanine transferase and aspartate transaminase are only moderately increased. The serum bilirubin level is usually normal early in the course of disease, but becomes elevated in most of the patients as the disease progresses. The immunofluorescence test for antimitochondrial antibodies (AMA) has a very high sensitivity, with numerous studies attesting to a positive rate of some 90–95% in histo-logically proven disease. Although the specificity of the test has not been systematically assessed, it is believed to fall well short of 100%. Recent work using recombinant autoantigens has resulted in the production of extremely reliable, sensitive and specific solid-phase tests (e.g. ELISA) for the detection of AMA (Leung et al, 1992; Moteki et al, 1996a).

Despite the sensitivity of serological testing, a confirmatory liver biopsy is usually required; it provides useful information on the stage of disease.

Radiological assessment of biliary patency by ultrasound or, in selected patients, by endoscopic retrograde cholangiopancreatography, is usually performed to exclude main bile-duct obstruction and gallstones. Difficulties in establishing the diagnosis arise when the serum levels of alkaline phosphatase is elevated and a test for AMA is positive in an asymptomatic patient. Although options differ, a liver biopsy in these circumstances can be recommended. The pathological changes in PBC are distinctively associated with the presence of widespread duct lesion, and the common scheme of histological grading of severity recognizes four stages (Dickson et al, 1979). In stage 1, a marker of early disease, small portal ductules show cellular damage and rupture, with bile leakage. There is also a dense periportal lymphoid infiltrate in which CD4$^+$ and CD8$^+$ T cells are found, together with monocytes, neutrophils, eosinophils and granuloma formation. In stage 2, piecemeal necrosis and/or proliferation of ductules are present. Stage 3 is marked by the presence of septal fibrosis and/or bridging necrosis, while stage 4 is typified by overt cirrhosis. In spite of the varying rates of histological progression among individual patients, 'primary biliary cirrhosis' is clearly a misnomer for a disease that has a long pre-cirrhotic stage. For this reason, the term 'autoimmune cholangiolitis' appears to more properly characterize this disease.

EPIDEMIOLOGY AND GENETIC PREDISPOSITION

PBC, while uncommon, is present among various ethnic and racial populations. Nonetheless, its incidence and prevalence vary quite widely, with highest levels found among Northern European populations (Galbraith et al, 1974; Salaspuro et al, 1976; Douglas and Finlayson, 1979) and at lower levels in Japan (Jaup and Zettergren, 1980; Sasaki et al, 1985), whereas the disease is almost non-existent in other parts of Asia. The anti-mitochondrial autoantibody response also varies within different ethnic groups, while the clinical manifestations of PBC appear similar among them (Table 1). Although these data could in part reflect the different availability of diagnostic tools and a fully trained hepatologist in communities, environmental factors are most likely to be involved. Even among populations derived from Northern European sources there is a striking difference in prevalence, with the highest reported prevalence found among inhabitants of regions of Northern England (Triger, 1980; Lofgren et al, 1985; Myszor and James, 1990). Of interest, in one study from Sheffield, United Kingdom, the prevalence of PBC cases in relation to one water reservoir appeared to be more than 10 times that of other reservoirs (Triger, 1980). Although results of water analysis were inconclusive, this study was extended for a further 10 years, and the original results were confirmed.

The reported existence of familial clustering of actual cases of PBC (Myszor and James, 1990), increased prevalence of various autoantibodies among relatives with PBC patients (Galbraith et al, 1974), and associations with class II histocompatibility antigens (Gores et al, 1987) indicate some

Table 1. Characteristic features of the antimitochondrial response in PBC.

	Autoantibody			
	PDC-E2	BCOADC-E2	OGDC-E2	E1α
Localization of the major B cell epitope	Inner lipoyl domain[a]	Inner lipoyl domain[b]	Inner lipoyl domain[c]	TPP binding site[d]
Amino acid residues	128–221	No distinct binding subregion	67–147	NA
Predominant Ig class and isotype	IgG3 and IgM[e]	NA	IgG2 and IgM[c]	NA
Inhibitory effect on the in vitro enzyme catalytic activity[f]	+	+	+	+
Percentage of reactivity according to ethnic background[g]				
Japanese	15/23 (65%)*	16/23 (70%)	11/23 (48%)	11/23 (47%)
American Caucasian	37/39 (95%)*	17/23 (73%)	12/39 (31%)	9/23 (39%)
Murine monoclonal antibodies				
V$_H$ gene usage[h]	Diverse array of V$_H$ gene segments	NA	NA	NA
Human combinatorial antibodies				
V$_H$ gene usage	Clonally related heavy chains displaying a high number of somatic mutations	NA	NA	NA

TPP = thiamine pyrophosphate. NA = not available.

* Statistically significant difference ($P = 0.0037$, Fisher's exact test).

[a] Surh et al (1990).
[b] Leung et al (1995).
[c] Moteki et al (1996b).
[d] Iwayama et al (1991).
[e] Surh et al (1988); Outschoorn et al (1993).
[f] van de Water et al (1988); Fregeau et al (1989); Sundin (1990); Uibo et al (1990).
[g] Iwayama et al (1992).
[h] Pascual et al (1994).

element, albeit low, of genetic risk for PBC. The assumption that PBC is an autoimmune disease has led to the search for genes within the major histocompatibility complex (MHC) which may be involved in predisposition to this disease. PBC has been associated with certain class II antigens of the MHC, including HLA-DR3, DR8, DR4 and DR2. In general, these earlier HLA correlations, based upon serological typing, were weak and varied considerably among reporting centres and different ethnic populations. More recently, molecular studies of MHC have provided more accurate methods for defining specific HLA alleles. Therefore, to define more precisely the role of the HLA class II genes in susceptibility of PBC, we have used the polymerase chain reaction (PCR) and sequence-specific oligonucleotide probes to type and compare the distribution of *DRB1*, *DQA1*, *DQB1* and *DPB1* in 51 Caucasian patients with PBC and 240 random Caucasian controls (Begovich et al, 1994). Although the allelic distribution at the *DPB1* locus showed no significant variation between patients and controls, there was heterogeneity in the distribution of DR–DQ haplotypes where the frequency of the *DRB1*0801-DQA1*0401/0601-DQB1*04* haplotype was significantly increased in patients, suggesting that it confers susceptibility to this disease. Two other haplotypes, *DRB1*1501-DQA1*0102-DQB1*0602* and *DRB1*1302-DQA1*0102-DQB1*0604*, were significantly reduced in patients, suggesting that they confer protection. Tests for the individual loci show that resistance to this disease is more strongly associated with the *DQA1*0102* allele shared by both protective haplotypes. Another attribute of HLA, linkage disequilibrium, adds an additional feature to the study of disease association with selective alleles. Instead of various alleles of each of these loci (e.g. *DRB1, DQB1* etc.) being randomly assorted on human chromosomes, various combinations of them occur more often than expected, especially in a given ethnic population (Arnett, 1995). Because these genes lie so close to one another, the finding of a particular allelic association with a disease does not imply that it is playing a direct role in the disease. Thus, it is unclear whether multiple genes or a single locus on the susceptible DR8 haplotype are needed for PBC predisposition. Nevertheless, these data suggest that distinct HLA class II alleles may play a role in the immunopathogenesis of this diseases by conferring both predisposition and resistance to PBC. Recently, Morling and colleagues (Morling et al, 1992) used restriction fragment polymorphism analysis to show that susceptibility to PBC in a Danish population was associated with the extended haplotype HLA-B8, DR3, *DQA1*0501, DQB1*0201*. Further studies in different ethnic groups (trans-racial gene mapping) are expected to define more precisely the most relevant PBC predisposing gene(s).

IMMUNOLOGICAL ASPECTS

In 1958, the detection of complement-fixing antibodies to tissue homogenates in the sera of a patient with PBC (Mackay, 1958), followed by the identification by indirect immunofluorescence of a distinct antimitochondrial staining pattern produced by PBC patients' sera (Walker et al, 1965; Berg et al, 1967), established for the first time the link between this disease and autoimmunity. The mitochondrial antibody reaction was soon found in clinical studies to have a high utility for the diagnostic identification of cases of PBC, whether tested for by complement fixation or immunofluorescence (Doniach et al, 1966; Goudie et al, 1966).

A decade later, antimitochondrial reactions other than that associated with PBC were successively described: either the mitochondrial antibody reaction differed in immunofluorescence characteristics or by chromato-graphic partition from that associated with PBC, or there was an accompanying disease that differed from PBC. The first such marker was the cardiolipin antigen utilized for serological tests of syphilis which had a mitochondrial location and was subsequently distinguished as M1 from the PBC-related antigen which was called M2 (Baum and Berg, 1981). Thereafter other putative mitochondrial antigens were reported and numbered M3 to M9; those associated with apparently variant forms of PBC became designated as M4, M8 and M9, and those associated with other diseases as M3, M5, M6 and M7 (Berg and Klein, 1986). Whereas the M1 and the M2 antigens are identifiable as cardiolipin and the pyruvate dehydrogenase complex respectively (see Table 2), the identity of the other mitochondrial autoantigens is in doubt (Palmer et al, 1993). Accordingly, it is suggested that the M3–M9 nomenclature be set aside pending clearer information on the character (if any) of these antigens and/or their disease associations (Davis et al, 1992). The mitochondrion is a complex organelle

Table 2. Mitochondrial autoantigens: molecular identity, earlier designation, molecular weight, function and frequency of the corresponding autoantibody in patients with PBC.

Subunits of the 2-oxo-acid dehydrogenase complex				
Molecular identity	Earlier designation[a]	Molecular weight (kDa)	Function	Autoantibody frequency (%)
PDH				
E1-α decarboxylase	M2d	41	Decarboxylates pyruvate with thiamine pyro-phosphate (TPP) as a co-factor	66
E1-β decarboxylase	M2e	36	Decarboxylase pyruvate with TPP as a co-factor	1–7
E2 acetyltransferase	M2a	74	Transfers acetyl group from E1 to coenzyme A (CoA)	92
Protein X	M2c	56	Unknown	NA
BCOADC				
E2 acyltransferase	M2c	52	Transfers acyl group from E1 to CoA	54
OGDC				
E2 succinyl transferase	M2c	48	Transfers succinyl group from E1 to CoA	66

[a] Nomenclature a–e as cited by Berg and Klein (1986).
PDH = pyruvate dehydrogenase; BCOADC = branched-chain 2-oxo-acid dehydrogenase; OGDC = 2-oxo-glutarate dehydrogenase.

that contains hundreds of proteins, including numerous enzymes of which some may well be autoantigenic. Nevertheless, a consensus should be reached with regard to the association between autoantibodies to such proteins with disease, before classification can be recommended.

In 1985 the new immunomolecular era for PBC began, initially with immunoblotting. This allowed the recognition of discrete polypeptide antigens of defined molecular weight (Figure 1) (Frazer et al, 1985). This was followed by the derivation by molecular cloning of a cDNA that encoded the major mitochondrial antigen for PBC (Gershwin et al, 1987), and thereafter the recognition of enzyme molecules of the 2-oxo-acid complexes as the reactants revealed by immunoblotting.

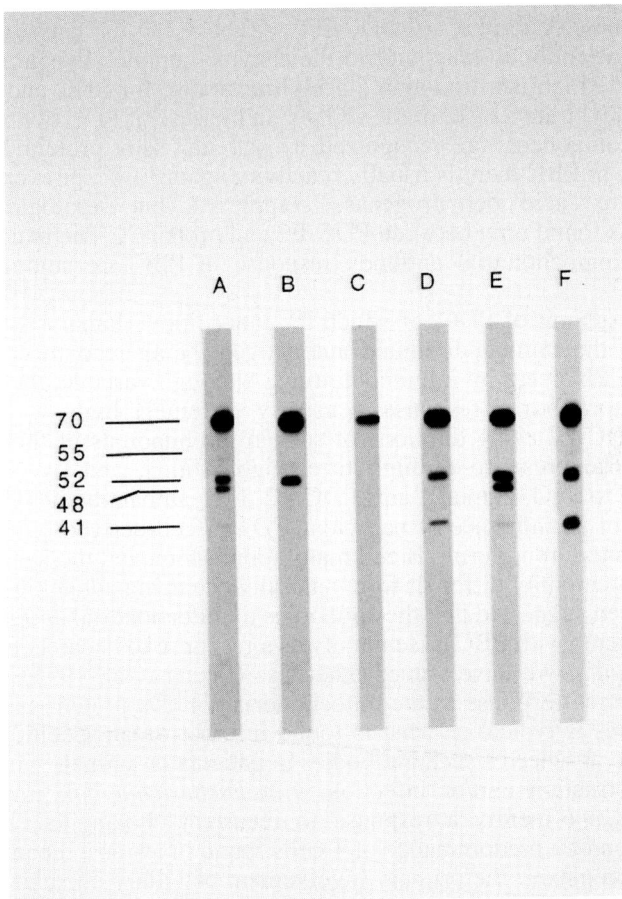

Figure 1. Immunoreactivity of PBC sera with beef heart mitochondria by Western blot showing different patterns of reactivity. Typical examples of PDC-E2 (70 kDa), protein X (55 kDa), BCOADC-E2 (52 kDa), OGDC-E2 (48 kDa) and E1α (41 kDa) reactivity are shown in lanes A–F.

Antimitichondrial autoantibodies

The presence of AMA is a major criterion for diagnosis of PBC. The titre of AMA does not correlate with the stages or prognosis of the disease, and whether or not these autoantibodies are involved in the pathogenesis of the disease remains unsettled. Nonetheless, antimitochondrial antibodies were the essential reagent that enabled the most critical recent development in the study of PBC: the cloning and subsequent identification of the target autoantigens in this disease (Gershwin et al, 1987). The mitochondrial autoantigens of PBC have been identified as components of a functionally related enzyme family, the 2-oxo-acid dehydrogenase complexes, which is located on the mammalian inner mitochondrial membrane and include the pyruvate dehydrogenase complex (PDC-E2), the branched-chain 2-oxo-acid dehydrogenase complex (BCOADC-E2) and the oxoglutarate dehydrogenase complex (OGDC-E2) (Table 2). In each case, the predominant antibody reactivity to the enzyme complex is against the E2 component which is a lipo-amide acetyltransferase for PDC and BOADC and a succinyl transferase for the OGDC. In the case of PDC two additional complex components are recognized by patients' sera: protein X and E1 (Figure 1). In PBC there is usually reactivity against two, or even all three of the 2-oxo-acid dehydrogenase complexes, but serological cross-reactivity is found only between PDC-E2 and protein X. The main features of the antimitochondrial antibody response in PBC are summarized in Table 2.

The E2 subunit of PDC, of which the inner lipoyl domain is the major epitope, is the immunodominant autoantigen, being recognized by over 90% of all PBC sera by immunoblotting. Although variable, the extent of the antimitochondrial response is usually extremely high, with specific titres to PDC-E2 using dilutions of sera in the hundreds of thousands or millions. The presence of high titre, high affinity, and overt subclass restriction to IgG3 among anti-PDC-E2 IgG autoantibodies is clearly indicative of an influence of particular CD4$^+$ T cell-derived lymphokines, such as γ-interferon, during B cell maturation. Moreover, the nature of this response is certainly different from naturally occurring autoantibodies.

It has been suggested that the antibodies to mitochondrial antigens in the sera of patients with PBC arise merely as a response to hepatocyte and bile ductular injury. We have argued otherwise (Leung et al, 1991). First, the highly directed response to the mitochondrial 74 kDa protein and the titre of antibodies is typical of what is found in other organ-specific diseases. Second, the absence of such antibodies in patients or animals with chronic biliary obstruction and/or infection with *Escherichia coli* implies that AMAs are not merely a response to recurrent cholangitis. Third, the constellation of a predominance of T cells found in lesions, the presence of immune complexes, the primary involvement of biliary ductular cells and the results of in vitro study of autoantibody production suggest that a target antigen is involved. Fourth, the similarities of the pathology of PBC to chronic graft-versus-host disease suggest that the injury is immunologically mediated.

Autoantibodies to non-mitochondrial targets, including various nuclear antigens, occasionally occur in some patients with PBC. The significance of these reactivities needs to be further addressed.

T cell response

The evidence that T cell response participates in the pathogenesis of PBC was initially derived from staining studies of histological samples and later by analysing lines that proliferate in the presence of putative mitochondrial autoantigens. The specificity of bile-duct destruction, together with the portal tract lymphoid infiltration and aberrant expression of HLA-DR molecules on biliary epithelium, suggests that intrahepatic biliary ductular epithelial cells themselves are direct targets of an intense and highly focused immune response (Nakanuma and Ohta, 1979; Yamada et al, 1986). In early lesions, CD8+ T lymphocytes are predominant, but an increased tendency towards CD4+ cells is observed in the advanced stages. However, it is still uncertain how these cells actually cause damage to ductular cells. The infiltrating T cells in PBC may be oligoclonal (Moebius et al, 1990), but cloning of autoreactive T cell lines from PBC has not been extensively explored.

In initial studies, we were able to derive antigen-specific autoreactive T cell clones from liver biopsies of patients with PBC, but not from livers affected with autoimmune hepatitis. The cloned T cell lines were specific for PDC-E2 and BCOADC-E2 as they produced interleukin 2 when stimulated with PDC-E2 and BCOADC-E2, but not with ovalbumin, tuberculin as PPD, or bovine gamma-globulin (BGG) (van de Water et al, 1991). More detailed data on cloned T cell lines have now been obtained by using T cell clones specific for PDC-E2 derived from both the liver and peripheral blood of patients with PBC (van de Water et al, 1995). The principal findings of these studies are summarized in Table 3. Interestingly, the reported T cell response differs from the B cell response in several ways. For PDC-E2 the most commonly recognized epitopic region by T cells was the outer lipoyl domain, whereas for the B cells it is the inner lipoyl domain (Table 1). The frequency of patients reactive to PDC-E2 was lower for T cells, but this may reflect the difficulties of the assay system. As the patients studied were in advanced stages of the disease process, some of the additional epitopes may have been recognized by responses elicited secondary to tissue damage by a process analogous to determinant spreading. Further observations involving patients at different stages of disease will help to clarify these interesting issues. Based on the concept that IL-2 and IFN-γ secretion is a property of Th1-like clones and IL-4 a property attributed to Th2-like clones, the lymphokine analysis in this study suggests that both T helper cell Th1- and Th2-like clones are present in the liver.

Of all cloned lines derived there were several CD4+/CD8+ line, but the vast majority of lines were CD4+. This is consistent with the lines being derived from patients late in the disease when CD4+ T cells in the liver are predominant. The presence of the CD4RO+ phenotype among isolated

Table 3. Autoreactive T cell clones specific for the E2 component of the pyruvate dehydrogenase complex in PBC.

PDC-specific T cell clones isolated from peripheral blood of PBC patients	Positive/total[a]
Proliferative response to PDC	16/19
Entire PDC complex	1/19
PDC-E2	10/19
PDC-E1	7/19[b]
Proliferative response to E2L1	6/11 (54%)[c]
Proliferating response to E2L2	4/11 (36%)

PDC-specific T cell clones isolated from the livers of PBC patients	
T cell phenotype	Predominance of CD4+ T cell lines
Lymphokine profile	IL-2, IL-4 and IFN-γ
T cell receptor phenotype	α/β
Vβ usage	Remarkable heterogeneity
CD45RO+	Positive/total
Patient 1	9/28 (32%)
Patient 2	2/23 (8.6%)

E2L1 = inner lipoyl domain; E2L2 = outer lipoyl domain.
[a] Positive to one or more mitochondrial antigens.
[b] Three of seven reactive patients reacted only to PDC-E1.
[c] Two of 11 patients responded to both E2L1 and E2L1.

clones indicates the presence of antigen-specific memory T cells in the liver. No satisfactory assay systems are currently available to assess the pathogenic capacity of these T cell lines, and this remains a major unsolved issue in PBC.

PATHOGENESIS

The current ability to clone and sequence autoantigens has permitted the search of protein data bases for similar sequences which occur in unrelated proteins of human, bacterial or viral origin. Molecular mimicry between host autoantigens and unrelated exogenous proteins, usually bacterial or viral, is one of the hypotheses used to explain how human autoantibodies to self proteins arise, break tolerance and lead to autoimmune disease (Horsfall, 1992). Examples of amino acid sequence homology among autoantigens include: the p70 (U1)RNP (Query and Keene, 1987) and topoisomerase I (Maul et al, 1989) with the p30[gag] retroviral nucleoprotein, the 60 kDa Ro/SS-A with the nuclear capsid of vesicular stomatitis virus (Scofield and Harley, 1991), fibrillarin with the nuclear protein encoded by Epstein–Barr virus, and the capsid protein P40 encoded by herpes virus type 1 (Kasturi et al, 1995). On the other hand, the presence of multiple B cell epitopes, characteristic of most autoantigens studied thus far, strongly supports the notion that the autoimmune response is driven by the antigen itself. These two theories are not necessarily contradictory, since the possibility of molecular mimicry at the level of a single epitope as the initiating event cannot be ruled out. For instance, McNeilage et al (1990) reported that, in Sjögren's syndrome, in the very early stage of the anti-SS-B/La response, only the N-terminal 107 amino acids are recognized, and, with time, the response broadens to include other epitopes. Interestingly, this region contains remarkable homology (amino acids 88–101) with an amino acid sequence in the gag protein of feline sarcoma virus (Kohsaka et al, 1990).

Molecular mimicry as a cause of PBC has been previously suggested, in part because of the highly conserved structure of PDC-E2, particularly its inner lipoyl domain, between bacteria, yeast and mammals. This thesis is strengthened by the fact that, for PDC-E2, in contrast to most of the known autoantigens, only a single extended B cell epitope in this conserved region has been identified. The bile ducts in PBC abnormally express class II HLA-DR and HLA-DQ antigens (Ballardini et al, 1984; Tsuneyama et al, 1995). Burroughs et al (1992) propose that the autoimmune phenomena in PBC result from T cell epitopes of microbial proteins being mimicked by peptides derived from, and presented by, the abnormally expressed HLA-DR antigen. Consistent with this hypothesis, Shimoda et al (1995) have recently demonstrated the presence of molecular mimicry at the T cell clonal level between human and E. coli PDC-E2. The reactivity of AMA with both human and bacterial mitochondria has also stimulated speculation that PBC may result from chronic bacterial infection (Stemerowicz et al, 1988) Indeed, chronic bacteriuria (Burroughs et al, 1984) and colonic infection with rough-colony (R) mutants of E. coli have been accorded significant pathogenic significance in PBC (Hopf et al, 1989). This scenario fails to explain why there is relatively weaker reactivity of PBC sera with bacterial 2-OADC enzymes compared with mammalian enzymes (Teoh et al, 1994). However, it may be argued that late in the disease, when self-tolerance has been lost, the continual exposure to self-antigen induces a secondary response of higher titre and affinity to the backbone peptide sequence. Studies using sera procured early in the disease process would help to resolve this issue.

Several studies have suggested that autoantigens relevant to PBC may be present on the surface of hepatocytes or biliary epithelium. PBC sera react with the surface of isolated hepatocytes and intact hepatoma cells; such reactivity is abolished by prior absorption of sera with mitochondria (Ghadiminejad and Baum, 1987). Sundin and Sundqvist (1991) detected reactivity of PBC sera with guinea-pig hepatocytes, and with 67- and 50-kDa components of isolated rat hepatocellular plasma membranes. Using rabbit sera specific to PDC-E2, Joplin and colleagues showed, in an immunohistochemical study, that cultured biliary epithelial cells from patients with PBC overexpress immunologically reactive material at the cell membrane (Joplin et al, 1995).

We have previously reported the development and characterization of PDC-E2 specific murine monoclonal antibodies, and human Fab monoclonal antibodies derived from a PBC lymph node Fab combinatorial library. Although most of them map to the inner lipoyl domain of PDC-E2, these antibodies exhibit distinct immunohistochemical characteristics. For instance, in immunofluorescent confocal microscope studies, two of these mAbs, the murine C355.1 and the human combinatorial SP1, demonstrate a distinct luminal staining pattern on bile duct epithelium (BDE) from patients with PBC, but not other control liver diseases (Figure 2) (van de Water et al, 1993). In contrast, all other mAbs produce only a typical cytoplasmic mitochondrial staining pattern on BDE and hepatocytes from PBC and control subjects. We believe that the observation that only a

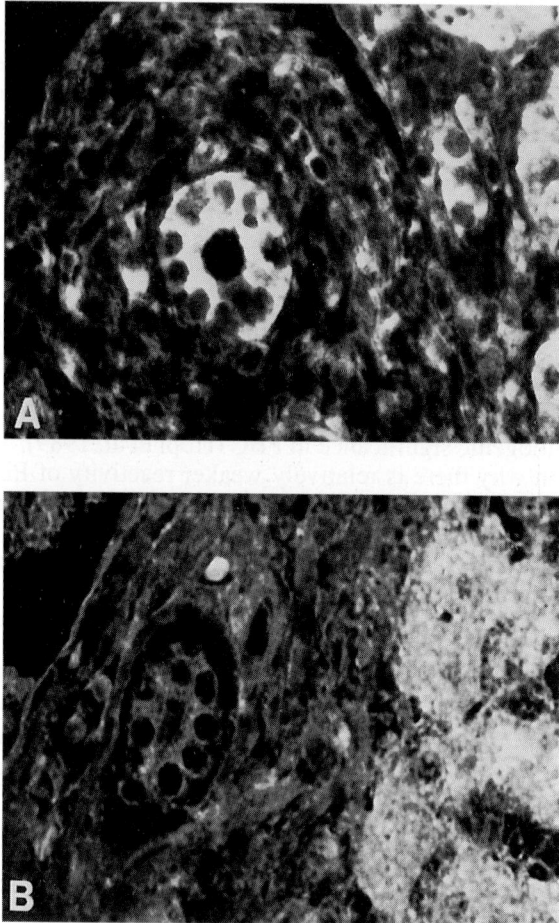

Figure 2. Confocal micrographs of liver sections stained with mAb C355.1. In (A), the PBC bile duct epithelium (BDE) shows intense homogeneous apical staining. In (B), the progressive sclerosing cholangitis BDE, studied at the same laser intensity for standardization, shows normal granular pattern typical of mitochondrial staining in the cytoplasm. In both liver sections mitochondrial staining in the cytoplasm of hepatocytes can be seen to the right of the bile duct.

selected number of anti-PDC-E2 reagents react with the apical region of BDE suggests that the elusive molecule targeted by these antibodies is a truncated or altered form of PDC-E2, or a cross-reactive molecule. Simultaneous examination of these sections with an anti-isotype reagent for human IgA revealed strong IgA staining in the luminal region of the BDE in patients with PBC; IgG and IgA antibodies to PDC-E2 were detected in the bile of patients with PBC but not normal controls.

To obtain insight into the nature of this elusive molecule, we use the PDC-E2 specific mAb C355.1 and human combinatorial SP1 described above to screen a random phage-epitope library expressing random dodeca-peptides. Eight different mimotope sequences with three common amino acid motifs (W-SYP, TYVS and VRH) were identified in 36 phage clones. Competitive inhibition of the immunohistochemical staining of PBC bile duct epithelium (BDE) was performed by incubating some of these peptides with C355.1, SP1 and control PDC-E2 specific murine and combinatorial antibodies. Interestingly, distinct peptides selectively inhibited C355.1 and SP1 unique luminal staining of PBC BDE, suggesting that such peptides might represent a mimotope of a cross-reactive molecule that exists primarily in the BDE of patients with PBC. Finally, using confocal microscopy, rabbit sera raised against a chosen mimotope peptide stained BDE from patients with PBC with higher intensity than controls. Comparable data were obtained with electron microscopy which, additionally, identified the molecule targeted by rabbit antisera as being located on the outer side of isolated BDE cells in PBC but not in normal controls. The mimotopes generated by these studies represent powerful reagents in the pressing need to identify the target molecule responsible for the luminal staining pattern observed when PBC BDE is stained with C355.1 and SP4.

The existence of this surface-expressed PDC-like molecule creates a compelling scenario in which the initial events in the pathogenesis of PBC would be a tissue-specific over expression of a novel substance with consequent presentation by class II MHC proteins aberrantly expressed on the PBC biliary ductular surface. This would allow induction of CD4$^+$ T cells that provide help for induction of CD8$^+$ cytotoxic cells. It is also possible that the PDC-E2-like neo-antigen may also be surface-expressed. A high level of intracellular expression of the neo-antigen would lead to an association with class I MHC molecules; reactivity against the biliary specific neo-antigen, perhaps by CD8$^+$ cytotoxic lymphocytes, would then lead to cell lysis and release of mitochondrial products. Presentation of released proteins to lymphocytes primed to the cross-reactive PDC-E2 could result in presentation of physically associated proteins such as other components of the PDC complex and synthesis of a wider range of auto-antibodies. It remains to be established to what degree the biliary epithelium is able to take over the function of a 'professional presenting cell' in a way that allows provision of the essential second signal such as that provided by the co-stimulatory molecule B7.

The exclusive presence of anti-PDC-E2 IgA in the bile of patients with PBC is also of further interest—in particular, the investigation of whether, during its transport, autoreactive IgA is capable of reacting with proteins in the biliary cell cytoplasm and thereby mediating metabolic dysfunctions that might result in cell death.

PROGNOSIS

The course in asymptomatic patients is variable and unpredictable. Some will never become symptomatic while others will run an inexorable and progressive deterioration course. By and large, the asymptomatic patient has, overall, the same life expectancy as other members of the population of the same age and sex and no therapy is indicated (Sherlock, 1994). Various prognostic models have been formulated, partially in order to allow timely identification of patients for which liver transplantation is indicated. Although some of them incorporate follow-up data in the development of the model, they are still limited by the lack of power to predict a life-threatening episode, such as bleeding oesophageal varices. Overall, a steadily rising level of serum bilirubin represents the best indication of deterioration. Low albumin, ascites, gastrointestinal bleeding, old age, low IgM, cirrhosis and central cholestasis constitute additional indicators of poor prognosis.

TREATMENT

There is still no satisfactory treatment for primary biliary cirrhosis. The thesis that PBC has an immunological basis has led to the use of immuno-suppressive and anti-inflammatory drugs in the treatment of this disease. The results, however, have been mostly discouraging or inconclusive. Corticosteroids, widely used in the past, do not favourably influence the natural history of the disease. Moreover, and particularly disappointing, corticosteroids do accelerate the progression of osteoporosis, an already serious problem in patients with primary biliary cirrhosis. D-Penicillamine has been extensively tested and abandoned because of toxicity and insignificant long-term benefit. Controlled prospective studies with azathioprine have yielded contradictory results but, in general, failed to show improvement in biochemistry or histology. Chlorambucil has been tested in a prospective, although unblinded, trial performed by the National Institute of Health in 24 patients followed by 2–6 years (Hoofnagle et al, 1986); an improvement in biochemical parameters and reduction in inflammatory infiltrate in liver biopsy was shown in the treated group but in association with a high incidence of bone marrow suppression and herpes infection. Cyclosporin A (CsA) may slow the progression of PBC, but clearly does not stop or reverse its course (Wiesner et al, 1990; Lombard et al, 1993). Furthermore, nephrotoxicity and hypertension associated with CsA administration represent an important constraint for its use (Minuk et al, 1988). In preliminary studies, a low dose of methotrexate (MTX) (15 mg/week) has been found to reduce pruritus, improve bio-chemical tests of liver function, and decrease the inflammation in portal triads (Kaplan, 1993). Nevertheless, the effect of MTX on survival is uncertain, and its use is not exempt from potentially harmful side-effects (Archna et al, 1994). Further randomized controlled trials are clearly needed to assess long-term benefits and safety. Colchicine, by virtue of its anti-inflammatory properties and impairment of collagen secretion, has also been used in an attempt to treat PBC. Safe and well tolerated, colchicine treatment has improved biochemistry data without improvement in symptoms or histology, although there is a suggestion that survival has improved (Kaplan et al, 1986; Bodenheimer et al, 1988; Warnes, 1991). However, the reported survival benefit from colchicine was small and was not confirmed in a long-term follow-up of one of the three randomized trials of colchicine (Zifroni and Schaffner, 1991).

Ursodeoxycholic acid (UDCA) has been one of the most scrutinized drugs in the treatment of PBC since the first favourable report by Poupon et al (1991). The effects of UDCA therapy have been attributed partially to its ability to change the bile-acid profile, with hydrophilic UDCA replacing more hydrophobic and considerably more hepatotoxic bile acids in the bile-acid pool. Although there have been indications that UDCA might have some in vitro immunomodulatory properties, this remains to be investigated more extensively. In the short-term controlled trial conducted by Poupon and colleagues, the use of UDCA significantly reduced levels of alkaline phosphatase, γ-glutamyltransferase, bilirubin and cholesterol, and slowed the rate of clinical deterioration in patients receiving this medication.

A number of subsequent small trials largely confirmed the effect on biochemical parameters of liver disease, but showed indeterminate effects on histological progression and treatment failure, including death and progression to liver transplantation. More recently, four double-blind placebo controlled trials were conducted in a significantly larger group of patients for at least 24 months (Table 4) (Heathcote et al, 1994; Lindor et al, 1994; Poupon et al, 1994; Combes et al, 1995). As with the majority of earlier, smaller trials, all four studies showed a clear beneficial effect of UDCA on the biochemical parameters of PBC, in particular the serum levels of bilirubin. In none of them, however, was UDCA able to reverse the disease process. Furthermore, these studies did not confirm the earlier optimism that this drug could significantly improve pruritus, one of the most distressing symptoms of the disease. Despite the considerable improvement in the design of these studies in comparison to the early trials, the critical issue of whether UDCA is able to slow disease progression remains unsolved. Although some histological improvement has been described, no significant differences were detected in progression to death between the UDCA and placebo groups in any of these four trials.

Liver transplantation has been highly successfully employed in PBC. Not only is the survival rate good following transplantation, but the majority of these patients are able to return to full-time employment (Scharschmidt, 1984; van Thiel et al, 1986). In the light of this, the lower rate of referral for liver transplant observed in one of the UDCA double-blind placebo-controlled trials (Poupon et al, 1994) should be cautiously

Table 4. Selected randomized, double-blind, placebo-controlled trials in the treatment of PBC.

	Number of patients	Duration of trial	Total daily dose	Improvement			End-point failures
				Symptoms[a]	Biochemical parameters[b]	Histological parameters	Development of cirrhosis and/or death
Ursodiol							
Lindor et al (1994)	108	Up to 4 years (mean follow-up: 2 years)	10–12 mg/kg	No	Yes	No	No difference from the placebo control group
Poupon et al (1994)	146	2 years	13–15 mg/kg	NA	Yes	NA	NA
Heathcote et al (1994)	222	2 years	14 mg/kg	No	Yes	↓ Frequency of progression of periportal hepatocellular ballooning and duct paucity	NA
Combes et al (1995)	151	2 years	13–15 mg/kg	No	Yes	↓ Frequency of progression of piecemeal necrosis, portal inflammation (stage 1), and fibrosis (stage 2)[c]	No difference from the placebo control group
Colchicine							
Kaplan et al (1986)	60	2 years	0.6 mg	No	Yes	No	↓ Mortality (?)
Zifroni and Schaffner (1991)	57	4 years	0.6 mg	No	Yes	No	No difference from the placebo control group
Cyclosporin A							
Wiesner et al (1990)	29	2 years	4.0 mg/kg	Yes	Yes	↓ Frequency of progression of portal inflammation	↓ Progression to cirrhosis
Lombard et al (1993)	349	6 years	3.0 mg/kg	Yes	Yes	No	↓ Mortality (?)

NA = not available.
[a] Fatigue and/or pruritus.
[b] At least bilirubin and alkaline phosphatase.
[c] As defined by Ludwig et al (1978).

interpreted. It is conceivable that this may reflect the fact that bilirubin levels, significantly lower in the UCDA-treated group, constitute an important criterion in the timing of referral for transplantation. What remains to be clarified is to what extent this decrease of bilirubin represents a true effect on the disease process rather than an independent consequence of the pharmacological effect of UDCA. This late possibility has fostered the suspicion that perhaps prolonged therapy with UDCA, and other presumably disease-modifying drugs, could in fact be detrimental for PBC patients. That would be the case if the reduction in bilirubin brought about by these drugs delays liver transplantation to the point at which the patients are too infirm or are in an age group for which this procedure would become less advisable on surgical grounds. In addition to evaluating biochemical parameters of cholestasis, further long-term trials should be designed to assess the effect of therapy on the symptoms and on the primary end points of death and transplantation.

It has been suggested that various combinations of UDCA, colchicine and methotrexate could represent a better alternative over either treatment alone (Kaplan, 1994). Nevertheless, until appropriate studies can evaluate the effectiveness and safety of this strategy, the combined use of these drugs cannot be recommended.

SUMMARY

Our understanding of the immunopathology of PBC has dramatically changed with the application of molecular biology techniques in clinical medicine. This has allowed, not only the possibility of characterizing mitochondrial autoantigens fully at the molecular level, but also the identification of specific sites on these molecules that are targetted by autoreactive B and T cells. In addition, the expression of cloned antigens has facilitated the development of the most reliable assays currently available for the detection of mitochondrial autoantibodies. The assessment of the pathogenic capacity of autoreactive T cells, as well as the characterization the PDC-E2 'look alike' molecule expressed on the cell membrane of PBC biliary epithelial cells, remain the major unsolved issues in this disease. Ideally, the continuous effort from both basic and clinical scientist in understanding the pathogenic mechanisms of PBC will lead to more specific, effective, and safer modalities of treatment.

REFERENCES

Archna S, Provenzale D, McKusick A et al (1994) Interstitial pneumonitits after low-dose methotrexate therapy in primary biliary cirrhosis. *Gastroenterology* **107:** 266–270.

Arnett FC (1995) HLA and autoimmunity in scleroderma (systemic sclerosis). *International Reviews in Immunology* **12:** 107–128.

Ballardini G, Bianchi FB, Doniach D et al (1984) Aberrant expression of HLA-DR antigens on bile duct epithelium in primary biliary cirrhosis: relevance to pathogenesis. *Lancet* **ii:** 1009–1013.

Baum H & Berg PA (1981) The complex nature of mitochondrial antibodies and their relation to primary biliary cirrhosis. *Seminars in Liver Disease* **1:** 309–321.

Begovich AB, Klitz W, Moonsamy PV et al (1994) Genes within the HLA class II region confer both predisposition and resistance to primary biliary cirrhosis. *Tissue Antigens* **43:** 71–77.

Berg PA & Klein R (1986) Mitochondrial antigens and autoantibodies: from anti-M1 to anti-M9. *Klinische Wochenschrift* **64:** 897–909.

Berg PA, Coniach D & Roitt IM (1967) Mitochondrial antibodies in primary biliary cirrhosis. I. Localization of the antigen to mitochondrial membranes. *Journal of Experimental Medicine* **126:** 227.

Bodenheimer H, Schaffner F & Pezzulo J (1988) Evaluation of colchicine therapy in primary biliary cirrhosis. *Gastroenterology* **95:** 124–129.

Burroughs AK, Rosenstein IJ, Epstein O et al (1984) Bacteriuria in primary biliary cirrhosis. *Gut* **25:** 133–137.

Burroughs AK, Sternberg MJE & Baum H (1992) Molecular mimicry in liver disease. *Nature* **358:** 377–378.

Combes B, Carithers RL Jr, Maddrey WC et al (1995) A randomized, double-blind, placebo-controlled trial of ursodeoxycholic acid in primary biliary cirrhosis. *Hepatology* **22:** 759–766.

Davis PA, Leung P, Manns M et al (1992) M4 and M9 antibodies in the overlap syndrome of primary biliary cirrhosis and chronic active hepatitis: epitopes or epiphenomena? *Hepatology* **16:** 1128–1136.

Dickson ER, Fleming CR & Ludwig J (1979). Primary biliary cirrhosis. In Popper H & Scaffner F (eds) *Progress in Liver Disease VI,* pp 487. New York: Grune & Stratton.

Doniach D, Roitt IM Walker JG et al (1966) Tissue antibodies in primary biliary cirrhosis, active chronic (lupoid) hepatitis, cryptogenic cirrhosis and other liver diseases and their clinical implications. *Clinical and Experimental Immunology* **1:** 237–262.

Douglas JG & Finlayson ND (1979) Are increased individual susceptibility and environmental factors both necessary for the development of primary biliary cirrhosis? *British Medical Journal* **2:** 419–420.

Frazer IH, Mackay IR, Jordan TW et al (1985) Reactivity of anti-mitochondrial autoantibodies in primary biliary cirrhosis: definition of two novel mitochondrial polypeptide autoantigens. *Journal of Immunology* **135:** 1739–1745.

Fregeau DR, Davis PA, Danner DJ et al (1989) Antimitochondrial antibodies of primary biliary cirrhosis recognize dihydrolipoamide acyltransferase and inhibit enzyme function of the branched chain alpha-ketoacid dehydrogenase complex. *Journal of Immunology* **142:** 3815–3820.

Galbraith RM, Smith M, Mackenzie RM et al (1974) High prevalence of seroimmunologic abnormalities in relatives of patients with chronic active hepatitis and prymary biliary cirrhosis. *New England Journal of Medicine* **290:** 63.

Gershwin ME, Mackay IR, Sturgess A et al (1987) Identification and specificity of a cDNA encoding the 70 kd mitochondrial antigen recognized in primary biliary cirrhosis. *Journal of Immunology* **138:** 3525–3531.

Ghadiminejad I & Baum H (1987) Reaction pattern of mitochondrial antibodies of primary biliary cirrhosis (PBC) is species specific but not organ specific. *Journal of Bioenergetics and Biomembranes* **19:** 239–253.

Gores GJ, Moore SB, Fischer LD et al (1987) Primary biliary cirrhosis: associations with class II major-histocompatibility complex antigens. *Hepatology* **7:** 889–892.

Goudie RB, Macsween RNM & Goldberg DM (1966) Serological and histological dignosis of primary biliary cirrhosis. *Journal of Clinical Pathology* **19:** 527–538.

Heathcote EJ, Cauch-Dudek K, Walker V et al (1994) The Canadian multicenter double-blind randomized controlled trial of ursodeoxycholic acid in primary biliary cirrhosis. *Hepatology* **19:** 1149–1156.

Hoofnagle JH, Davis GL, Schafer DF et al (1986) Randomized trial of chlorambucil for primary biliary cirrhosis. *Gastroenterology* **91:** 1327–1334.

Hopf U, Moller B, Stemerowicz R et al (1989) Relation between *Escherichia coli* R(rough)-forms in gut, lipid A in liver, and primary biliary cirrhosis. *Lancet* **ii:** 1419–1422.

Horsfall AC (1992) Molecular mimicry and autoantigens in connective tissue disease. *Molecular Biology Reports* **16:** 39–47.

Iwayama T, Leung PSC, Coppel RL et al (1991) Specific reactivity of recombinant human PDC-Ela in primary biliary cirrhosis. *Journal of Autoimmunity* **4:** 769–778.

Iwayama T, Leung PS, Rowley M et al (1992) Comparative immunoreactive profiles of Japanese and

American patients with primary biliary cirrhosis against mitochondrial autoantigens. *International Archives of Allergy and Immunology* **99**: 28–33.

Jaup BH & Zettergren LSW (1980) Familial occurrence of primary biliary cirrhosis associated with hypergamaglobulinemia in descendants: a family study. *Gastroenterology* **78**: 549–555.

Joplin R, Wallace LL, Johnson GD et al (1995) Subcellular localization of pyruvate dehydrogenase dihydrolipoamide acetyltransferase in human intrahepatic biliary epithelial cells. *Journal of Pathology* **176**: 381–390.

Kaplan MM (1993) New strategies needed for treatment of primary biliary cirrhosis? (editorial). *Gastroenterology* **104**: 651–653.

Kaplan MM (1994) Primary biliary cirrhosis—a first step in prolonging survival (editorial). *New England Journal of Medicine* **330**: 1386–1387.

Kaplan MM, Alling DW, Zimmerman HJ et al (1986) A prospective trial of colchicine for primary biliary cirrhosis. *New England Journal of Medicine* **315**: 1448–1454.

Kasturi KN, Hatakeyama A, Spiera H et al (1995) Antifibrillarin autoantibodies present in systemic sclerosis and other connective tissue diseases interact with similar epitopes. *Journal of Experimental Medicine* **181**: 1027–1036.

Kohsaka H, Yamamoto K, Fujii H et al (1990) Fine epitope mapping of the human SS-B/La protein. Identification of a distinct autoepitope homologous to a viral gag polyprotein. *Journal of Clinical Investigation* **85**: 1566–1574.

Leung PSC, van de Water J, Coppel RL et al (1991) Molecular characterization of the mitochondrial autoantigens in primary biliary cirrhosis. *Immunologic Research* **10**: 518–527.

Leung PSC, Iwayama T, Prindiville T et al (1992) Use of designer recombinant mitochondrial antigens in the diagnosis of primary biliary cirrhosis. *Hepatology* **15**: 367–372.

Leung PS, Chuang DT, Wynn RM et al (1995) Autoantibodies to BCOADC-E2 in patients with primary biliary cirrhosis recognize a conformational epitope. *Hepatology* **22**: 505–513.

Lindor KD, Dickson ER, Baldus WP et al (1994) Ursodeoxycholic acid in the treatment of primary biliary cirrhosis. *Gastroenterology* **106**: 1284–1290.

Lofgren J, Jarnerot G, Danielsson D et al (1985) Incidence and prevalence of primary biliary cirrhosis in a defined population in Sweden. *Scandinavian Journal of Gastroenterology* **20**: 647–650.

Lombard M, Portmann B, Neuberger J et al (1993) Cyclosporin A treatment in primary biliary cirrhosis: results of a long-term placebo controlled trial. *Gastroenterology* **104**: 519–526.

Ludwig J, Dickson ER & McDonald GS (1978) Staging of chronic nonsuppurative destructive cholangitis (syndrome of primary biliary cirrhosis). *Virchows Archiv A: Pathologie Pathologische Anatomie* **379**: 103–112.

Mackay IR (1958) Primary biliary cirrhosis showing a high titer of autoantibody. *New England Journal of Medicine* **258**: 185.

McNeilage LJ, Macmillan EM & Whittingham SF (1990) Mapping of epitopes on the La (SS-B) autoantigen of primary Sjögren's syndrome: identification of a cross-reactive epitope. *Journal of Immunology* **145**: 3829–3835.

Maul GG, Jimenez SA, Riggs E et al (1989) Determination of an epitope of the diffuse systemic sclerosis marker antigen DNA topoisomerase I: sequence similarities with retroviral p30 gag protein suggests a possible cause for autoimmunity in systemic sclerosis. *Proceedings of the National Academy of Sciences of the USA* **86**: 8492–8496.

Minuk GY, Bohme CE, Burgess E et al (1988) Pilot study of cyclosporin A in patients with primary biliary cirrhosis. *Gastroenterology* **95**: 1356–1363.

Moebius U, Manns M, Hess G et al (1990) T-cell receptor gene rearrangements of lymphocytes—T infiltrating the liver in chronic hepatitis B and primary biliary cirrhosis (PBC) oligoclonality of PBC-derived T cell clones. *European Journal of Immunology* **20**: 889–896.

Morling N, Dalhoff K, Fugger L et al (1992) DNA polymorphism of HLA class II genes in primary biliary cirrhosis. *Immunogenetics* **35**: 112–116.

Moteki S, Leung PSC, Dickson ER et al (1996a) Use of a designer triple expression hybrid clone for three different lipoyl domains for the detection of antimitochondrial antibodies. *Hepatology* (in press).

Moteki S, Leung PSC, Dickson ER et al (1996b) Epitope mapping and reactivity of autoantibodies to the E2 component of 2-oxoglutarate dehydrogenase complex in primary biliary cirrhosis using recombinant 2-oxoglutarate dehydrogenase complex. *Hepatology* **23**: 436–444.

Myszor M & James OFW (1990) The epidemiology of primary biliary cirrhosis in England: an increased common disease? *Quarterly Journal of Medicine* **75**: 377–385.

Nakanuma Y & Ohta G (1979) Histometric and serial observations of the intrahepatic bile ducts in primary biliary cirrhosis. *Gastroenterology* **76:** 1326–1332.

Outschoorn I, Rowley MJ, Cook AD et al (1993) Subclasses of immunoglobulins and autoantibodies in autoimmune diseases. *Clinical Immunology and Immunopathology* **66:** 59–66.

Palmer JM, Yeaman SJ, Bassendine, MF et al (1993) M4 and M9 autoantigens in primary biliary cirrhosis—a negative study. *Journal of Hepatology* **18:** 251–254.

Pascual V, Cha S, Gershwin ME et al (1994) Nucleotide sequence analysis of natural and combinatorial anti-PDC-E2 antibodies in patients with primary biliary cirrhosis. Recaptulating immune selection with molecular biology. *Journal of Immunology* **152:** 2577–2585.

Poupon RE, Balkau B, Eschwege E et al (1991) A multicenter, controlled trial of ursodiol for the treatment of primary biliary cirrhosis. *New England Journal of Medicine* **324:** 1548–1554.

Poupon RE, Poupon R & Balkau B (1994) Ursodiol for the long-term treatment of primary biliary cirrhosis. The UDCA-PBC Study Group. *New England Journal of Medicine* **330:** 1342–1347.

Query CC & Keene JD (1987) A human autoimmune protein associated with U1 RNA containing a region of homology that is cross-reactive with retroviral p30 gag antigen. *Cell* **51:** 211–220.

Salaspuro MP, Laitinen OI, Lehtola J et al (1976) Immunological parameters, viral antibodies, and biochemical and histological findings in relatives of patients with chronic active hepatitis and primary biliary cirrhosis. *Scandinavian Journal of Gastroenterology* **11:** 313–320.

Sasaki H, Inoue K, Higuchi K et al (1985) Primary biliary cirrhosis in Japan: national survey by the subcommittee on autoimmune hepatitis. *Gastroenterologia Japonica* **20:** 476–485.

Scharschmidt BF (1984) Human liver transplantation: analysis of data on 540 patients from four centers. *Hepatology* **4 (supplement):** 95S.

Scofield RH & Harley JB (1991) Autoantigenicity of Ro/SSA antigen related to a nucleocapsid protein of vesicular stomatitis virus. *Proceedings of the National Academy of Sciences of the USA* **88:** 3343–3347.

Sepersky R, Callow A, Kanel G et al (1982) Portasystemic shunts in primary biliary cirrhosis: survival is the same as in patients with Laennec's cirrhosis and postnecrotic cirrhosis. *Digestive Diseases and Sciences* **27:** 507–512.

Sherlock S (1994) Primary biliary cirrhosis: clarifying the issues. *American Journal of Medicine* **96 (supplement 1A):** 27S–33S.

Shimoda S, Nakamura M, Ishibashi H et al (1995) HLA DRB4 0101-restricted immunodominant T cell autoepitope of pyruvate dehydrogenase complex in primary biliary cirrhosis: evidence for molecular mimicry in human autoimmune diseases. *Journal of Experimental Medicine* **181:** 1835–1845.

Spinsi R, Smith-Laing G, Epstein O et al (1981) Results of portal decompression in patients with primary biliary cirrhosis. *Gut* **22:** 345–349.

Stemerowicz R, Hopf U, Moller B et al (1988) Are antimitochondrial antibodies in primary biliary cirrhosis induced by R(rough)-mutants of enterobacteriaceae? *Lancet* **ii:** 1166–1170.

Sundin U (1990) Antibody binding and inhibition of pyruvate dehydrogenase (PDH) in sera from patients with primary biliary cirrhosis. *Clinical and Experimental Immunology* **81:** 238.

Sundin U & Sundqvist KG (1991) Plasma membrane association of primary biliary cirrhosis mitochondrial marker antigen M2. *Clinical and Experimental Immunology* **83:** 407–412.

Surh CD, Cooper AE, Coppel RL et al (1988) The predominance of IgG3 and IgM isotype antimitochondrial antibodies against recombinant fused mitochondrial peptide in patients with PBC. *Hepatology* **8:** 290–295.

Surh CD, Coppel R & Gershwin ME (1990) Structural requirement for autoreactivity on human pyruvate dehydrogenase-E2, the major mitochondrial autoantigen in primary biliary cirrhosis. *Journal of Immunology* **144:** 3367–3374.

Teoh KL, Mackay IR, Rowley MJ et al (1994) Enzyme inhibitory antibodies to pyruvate dehydrogenase complex in primary biliary cirrhosis differ for mammalian, yeast and bacterial enzymes: implications for molecular mimicry. *Hepatology* **19:** 1029–1033.

Triger DR (1980) Primary biliary cirrhosis: an epidemiological study. *British Journal of Medicine* **281:** 772–775.

Tsuneyama K, van de Water J, Leung PSC et al (1995) Abnormal expression of PDC-E2 on the luminal surface of biliary epithelium occurs before MHC class II and BB1/B7 expression. *Hepatology* **21:** 1031–1037.

Uibo R, McKay IR, Rowley M et al (1990) Inhibition of enzyme function by human autoantibodies to an autoantigen pyruvate dehydrogenase E2: different epitope for spontaneous human and induced rabbit autoantibodies. *Clinical and Experimental Immunology* **80:** 19.

van de Water J, Fregeau D, Davis P et al (1988) Autoantibodies of primary biliary cirrhosis recognize dihydrolipoamide acetyltransferase and inhibit enzyme function. *Journal of Immunology* **141:** 2321–2324.

van de Water J, Ansari AA, Surh CD et al (1991) Evidence for the targeting by 2-oxo-dehydrogenase enzymes in the T cell response of primary biliary cirrhosis. *Journal of Immunology* **146:** 89–94.

van de Water J, Turchany J, Leung PS et al (1993) Molecular mimicry in primary biliary cirrhosis. Evidence for biliary epithelial expression of a molecule cross-reactive with pyruvate dehydrogenase complex-E2. *Journal of Clinical Investigation* **91:** 2653–2664.

van de Water J, Ansari A, Prindiville T et al (1995) Heterogeneity of autoreactive T cell clones specific for the E2 component of the pyruvate dehydrogenase complex in primary biliary cirrhosis. *Journal of Experimental Medicine* **181:** 723–733.

van Thiel DH, Tarter R & Gavaler JS (1986) Liver transplantation in adults: an analysis of costs and benefits at the University of Pittsburg. *Gastroenterology* **90:** 211–216.

Walker JG, Doniach D, Roitt IM et al (1965) Serological tests in diagnosis of primary biliary cirrhosis. *Lancet* **i:** 827.

Warnes TW (1991) Colchicine in primary biliary cirrhosis. *Alimentary Pharmacology and Therapeutics* **5:** 321–329.

Wiesner RH, Ludwig J, Lindor KD et al (1990) A controlled trial of cyclosporine in the treatment of primary biliary cirrhosis. *New England Journal of Medicine* **322:** 1419–1424.

Yamada G, Hyodo I, Tobe K et al (1986) Ultrastructural immunocytochemical analysis of lymphocytes infiltrating bile duct epithelia in primary biliary cirrhosis. *Hepatology* **6:** 385–391.

Zifroni A & Schaffner F (1991) Long-term follow-up of patients with primary biliary cirrhosis on colchicine therapy. *Hepatology* **14:** 990–993.

6

Immunopathogenesis of viral hepatitis

BARBARA REHERMANN

Viral hepatitis is an inflammatory disease of the liver which can be caused by a variety of distinct infectious agents. So far, the hepatitis A, B, C, D and E viruses and, most recently, the hepatitis GB viruses A, B and C, the latter also termed hepatitis G virus, have been identified. More than 500 million people world-wide are infected, and the spectrum of disease ranges from acute self-limited to chronic hepatitis which eventually causes severe life-threatening complications such as liver cirrhosis and hepatocellular carcinoma. This whole spectrum of disease not only reflects the different biological properties and pathogenicity of the hepatitis viruses, but is also the result of the specific interaction between each virus and the immune system of the infected host. The immune response plays a crucial role both for the elimination of the virus and resolution of disease, on the one hand, and for disease pathogenesis, i.e. liver injury, on the other hand.

This chapter describes the characteristics of a successful immune response able to resolve acute hepatitis and to guarantee lasting protection against recurrence of disease or re-infection, characterizes the pathogenetic role of the immune response during chronic hepatitis, analyses mechanisms of viral persistence and discusses new immunomodulatory therapies for viral hepatitis.

THE HEPATITIS VIRUSES

One way to group the hepatitis viruses is by their route of transmission. An enteral, i.e. faecal–oral route of transmission is characteristic for the hepatitis A and E viruses. The hepatitis A virus is a picornavirus of 27 nm (Lemon et al, 1994) and the hepatitis E virus is an RNA virus of similar size (27–30 nm) which is closely related to the calicivirus family (Krawczynski and Bradley, 1989; Tam et al, 1991). Both of these viruses can cause acute hepatitis, in the case of HEV infection of pregnant women even fatal hepatitis, but are never associated with chronic hepatitis and liver cirrhosis.

Parenterally transmitted viruses are the hepatitis B, C and D viruses and the group of recently identified GB viruses. With the exception of the

Baillière's Clinical Gastroenterology—
Vol. 10, No. 3, September 1996
ISBN 0–7020–2187–3
0950–3528/96/030483 + 18 $12.00/00

hepatitis D virus, which depends on the envelope proteins of the hepatitis B virus to maintain its life cycle, this group consists of the main agents responsible for blood transfusion-associated hepatitis. Although they are all capable of inducing acute as well as chronic hepatitis and hepatocellular carcinoma, their molecular and biological characteristics differ considerably.

The hepatitis B virus (HBV) is a small, non-cytopathic virus with a circular DNA genome of approximately 3200 nucleotides, which encodes several envelope (preS1, preS2, HBsAg), nucleocapsid (HBcAg, HBeAg), transactivating (X) and polymerase (Pol) proteins (Tiollais et al, 1985).

The hepatitis C virus on the other hand consists of a positive-stranded RNA genome of approximately 9400 nucleotides, is smaller than 80 nm and is related to the group of togae and flaviviridae. It encodes a polyprotein of 3010–3011 amino acids, which is cleaved post- and co-translationally by proteases encoded by the viral genome itself and by the host (Choo et al, 1989).

The newly identified GB viruses GBV-A and B are closely related to HCV, as is evident from an amino acid sequence homology of 47–57% of the putative RNA helicase. As is the case in HCV, these two viruses have positive-stranded, linear RNA genomes of approximately 10 kb in length with structural proteins at the 5′ end and non-structural proteins at the 3′ end. GBV-C displays a high degree of similarity with GBV-A, i.e. 59% at the nucleotide level and 64% at the amino acid level (Leary et al, 1996).

As different as the biological characteristics of these parenterally transmitted viruses are the clinical courses of disease they induce. Hepatitis B virus infection of immunocompetent adults usually manifests as an acute illness which is followed by clinical recovery and viral clearance in 90% of the cases. Vertical transmission of the hepatitis B virus, i.e. from mother to newborn, however, results in persistent infection and chronic hepatitis later on in life. This route of transmission accounts for the majority of hepatitis B virus infections world-wide, mainly in highly populated areas such as Asia and Africa.

In contrast to HBV infection, HCV infection is most often clinically inapparent and rarely associated with symptoms of acute hepatitis. Accordingly, in almost 40% of infected patients, the time point and route of infection are not known. Many patients, however, fail to resolve the acute infection and proceed to develop chronic hepatitis, liver cirrhosis and hepatocellular carcinoma (Choo et al, 1989; Alter et al, 1992).

Finally, the GB viruses, which were first detected in a surgeon with non-A non-B hepatitis, and were shown to induce severe hepatitis in tamarins, are found mainly in co-infections together with HBV or HCV. Although they can cause acute as well as chronic hepatitis, the most striking observation is that 1–2% of apparently healthy volunteer blood donors have been found to display antibodies against these viruses (Simons et al, 1995). The reason for the high prevalence of persistent infections without apparent liver disease is unclear at this time. The following chapter describes the components of an antiviral immune response in general and exemplifies its role in HBV and HCV infection, which have been studied in detail.

COMPONENTS OF THE ANTIVIRAL IMMUNE RESPONSE

While the mechanisms leading to hepatitis, chronic liver disease and hepatocellular carcinoma are not well understood, it is likely that both direct mechanisms, unique to each of these parenterally transmitted viruses, and indirect mechanisms, reflecting the effects of an antiviral immune response, play a causative role in the outcome of disease. Unfortunately, studies aimed at analysing direct cytopathic effects of each of these viruses have so far been hampered by the fact that the host-range of the viruses is limited and that appropriate in vitro culture systems are not available. On the other hand, several clinical observations support the notion that the infected host's immune response not only contributes to the resolution of disease and protection of the host, but also to disease pathogenesis and liver cell injury. The main argument is that persistent infection without evidence of liver cell injury is frequent for both hepatitis B and C virus infection if the host is immunosuppressed or immunologically immature (Hollinger, 1990). For example, the percentage of chronic HBV infection is increased to 30–80% in patients undergoing haemodialysis (Szmuness et al, 1974; Degos et al, 1988) or chemotherapy (Wands et al, 1974) and in patients suffering from Down's syndrome or HIV infection (McDonald et al, 1987; Brook et al, 1989; Hadler et al, 1991). Morever, it is generally estimated that the speed of hepatitis B virus elimination decreases after the age of 40 (Archer et al, 1983) and that the development of a carrier state is favoured after the age of 60 (Nishihara, 1983) due to a decreased immune response state. Hence, most HBV infections at the beginning and end of life do not resolve, but result in chronic liver disease.

The following paragraphs will outline the kinetics and quality of virus–host interaction which contribute to the course and long-term outcome of disease.

In the earliest phase of any viral infection, viral factors such as size and route of the inocculum, as well as the speed of replication, determine the rate at which host cells become infected. This process is opposed by non-specific immune defence mechanisms such as the NK cell system (Moretta et al, 1994). Simultaneously, or soon after, virus-specific immunity is induced by antigen-presenting cells such as dendritic cells and macrophages that process and present viral antigens to T and B lymphocytes in the regional lymph nodes. Specifically, the interaction of virus-specific T helper cells with B cells and cytotoxic T cells forms the antiviral immune response.

T helper cells play a central immunoregulatory role. The specifically rearranged T cell receptor of these CD4+ cells recognizes peptide fragments which have been proteolytically cleaved from endogenously processed antigens and are then displayed by HLA class II molecules on the cell membrane of antigen-presenting cells. The CD4+ T cell response exerts regulatory functions (Vitetta et al, 1989) by providing help to antigen-specific CD8+ cells (Doherty et al, 1992) and B cells. First, they regulate the induction of cytotoxic T cells via differential secretion of cytokines. In HIV infection, it has been reported that the cytokine profile of T helper 1 cells

(IL-2, γ IFN, TNFα) favours resolution of infection, while a different set of cytokines secreted by T helper 2 cells (IL-4, IL-5, IL-10) induces progression of disease. Whether these mechanisms play an identical role in hepatitis virus infection is still unproven, and may be different for each of the viruses. Second, cytokines such as γIFN and TNFα which can be produced by CD4[+] cells have been shown to exert direct antiviral effects in hepatitis B virus infection. Specifically, HBV gene expression in infected hepatocytes is down-regulated to an undetectable level (Guidotti et al, 1994a,b). This process could obviously represent a very efficient antiviral defence mechanism in the infected host. However, it has only been shown in hepatitis B virus, not in hepatitis C virus infection, and at this time it is unclear whether this is due to an inappropriate cytokine production of HCV-specific CD4[+] cells or due to a unique non-responsiveness of the hepatitis C virus. Finally, CD4[+] T cells have also been reported to exert cytotoxic functions and even to be able to kill virus-antigen presenting CD8[+] cells in vitro (Franco et al, 1992). While the physiological significance of this cytotoxic effect against virus-infected cells has not been explored in vivo, it might represent an important regulatory loop able to limit the immune response to the virus.

The immune response of CD8[+] T cells represents another main effector limb during viral infection. These cells recognize endogenously synthesized peptides presented in the antigen-binding groove of HLA class I molecules on the surface of virus-infected cells. HLA class I–peptide interactions are allele-specific in the sense that the peptide must be between eight and 11 amino acids long and contain an HLA allele-specific binding motif determined by the second amino acid from the amino terminus and the last amino acid at the carboxy terminus. Peptide-activated CD8[+] T cells then kill virus infected hepatocytes by induction of apoptosis or lysis. Recent evidence indicates that these cells can also clear HBV without harming the infected cell by a cytokine-mediated mechanism (Gilles et al, 1992; Guidotti et al, 1994a,b).

ACUTE, SELF-LIMITED HEPATITIS: MECHANISMS OF VIRAL CLEARANCE

Hepatitis B

One of the most interesting and clinically relevant issues of current research is the question: under which circumstances does an acute viral hepatitis resolve, and under which conditions does it progress to chronic liver disease? Most experimental data which could contribute to an answer of this question have been obtained from hepatitis B virus-infected immuno-competent adults. Patients who are able to resolve an acute hepatitis B virus infection are characterized by a distinct humoral and cellular immune response that clearly distinguishes them from patients with chronic liver disease. As far as the humoral immune response is concerned, antibodies are targeted against all proteins of the infectious HBV virion, the 42 nm

Dane particle, which consists of a lipoprotein envelope containing three envelope polypeptides and a nucleocapsid, formed by the hepatitis core antigen, the HBV polymerase and the HBV genome. While all antibodies are able to form immune complexes with free viral particles, which are then complexed, phagocytosed by antigen-presenting cells and processed efficiently for presentation to T cells, not all of them are protective.

Certain antibody patterns have been recognized during the natural course of hepatitis B and have therefore been used as diagnostic tools to distinguish acute, resolved and chronic forms of HBV infection. The first markers in acute hepatitis B are antibodies against the core antigen which are not lost, even if the virus is cleared later on. Their life-long production might be explained by the fact that they are the only antibodies that can be produced without T cell help. Antibodies against the carboxy-terminus and especially against the RNase H domain of the polymerase (Feitelson et al, 1988; Chang et al, 1989; Weimer et al, 1989; Yuki et al, 1990), an early protein during HBV replication, are detectable early in the infection as well (Weimer et al, 1990).

Anti-HBe antibodies are an early sign of recovery associated with a significant decrease of viral replication, loss of HBe antigen and less severe liver disease. Anti-HBs antibodies are associated with the final resolution of disease. They are targeted against two domains between amino acid positions 124 and 147 (Ashton-Rickardt and Murray, 1989) which form the 'a' determinant common to all HBV subtypes and confer, in most cases, protective immunity against re-infection. Interestingly, a few vaccine-induced escape mutants with high replication levels despite antiHBs antibodies, have been described, which encode arginine in place of glycine at position 145 due to a G-to-A point mutation (Carmen et al 1990; Harrison et al, 1991). This larger and charged residue changes the hydrophobicity profile of the second loop of the 'a' determinant, supposedly also changing the secondary and tertiary structure of the antigen and altering the epitope recognition by anti-HBs antibodies (Waters et al, 1992). Carriers of these HBV escape mutants may therefore transmit HBV by donation of blood units without detectable surface antigen to recipients, even if the latter are vaccinated.

At the same time or even prior to the humoral immune response, a cellular immune response is mounted by patients with acute, self-limited viral hepatitis. This immune response consists of a polyclonal HLA class I- and class II-restricted T cell response against multiple HBV encoded antigens.

As far as the HLA class II-restricted immune response of CD4[+] T cells is concerned, the nucleocapsid antigens seem to be recognized most efficiently. The epitopes recognized on HBcAg are located primarily between amino acid positions 1–20, 50–69 and 117–131 (Ferrari et al, 1991). There is evidence that the proliferative T cell response to HBcAg coincides with seroconversion and clearance of viral antigen from the serum. It is thought that these nucleocapsid-specific T cells probably stimulate HBV-specific B cells to produce neutralizing anti-HBs antibodies.

Similar to the class II-restricted T cell response, most patients with acute hepatitis B who are able to clear the infection mount a vigorous HLA class I-restricted T cell response that is readily detectable in the peripheral blood, whereas chronically infected patients do not. Most interestingly, the CD4+ and CD8+ T cell response seems to persist for decades after recovery from acute hepatitis B and seems to protect from viral re-infection and from re-activation of hepatitis. Patients studied for up to 30 years after recovery from acute hepatitis B virus infection and antigen clearance, maintained a multispecific CTL response targeted against many different proteins and the immune response correlated with the presence or absence of HBV DNA in serum or lymphocytes (Rehermann et al, 1995a). HBV is probably transcriptionally active in these patients because it co-exists with, and appears actively to maintain a CTL response. Cytotoxic T cells display the phenotype of recently activated cells, i.e. the activation markers DR and CD69 on their surface, indicating recent antigen contact, and their precursor frequency remains at nearly acute-stage levels for many years. These findings suggest that minute traces of replicating virus seem to actively maintain a CTL response, and vice versa are held in cheek by the co-existing CTL.

While immunocompetent adult patients with acute hepatitis B usually produce a strong CTL response to HBV and eliminate the virus, patients with chronic HBV infection generally show a weak or undetectable peripheral blood CTL response. Nonetheless, antigen-specific CD8+ T cells can be isolated and expanded from the liver of patients with chronic infection, but it appears that they are present at much lower frequencies than in the livers of patients with acute hepatitis (Barnaba et al, 1989). Overall, the disease activity seems to correlate with the degree of the T cell response. In this respect, exacerbations of disease have been shown to be preceded by increased CD4+ cell activity (Tsai et al, 1992). Similarly, CD8+ cells, which have been demonstrated at very low frequency in the blood of patients with chronic hepatitis B, can be activated and expanded in those patients who experience spontaneous or interferon-mediated induction of HBe- and HBs-specific antibodies and resolution of disease (Rehermann et al, 1996). In some of those patients the number of HBV-specific CTL precursors in the peripheral blood is as high as it is after clearance of acute infection, suggesting that resolution of acute as well as chronic hepatitis is based on the same immunological mechanisms and that it may be induced by enhancement of the cellular immune response.

In both settings, i.e. resolution of acute as well as chronic hepatitis, viral clearance is profound but not absolute because minute traces of HBV DNA are still detectable in serum and/or in lymphocytes of individual patients. The data suggest that the hepatitis B virus is controlled by the cellular and humoral immune response rather than being completely eradicated after resolution of acute and chronic hepatitis B infection.

Since DNA sequence analysis revealed that epitope mutations did not account for viral persistence in these patients (Rehermann et al, 1995a), it is possible that the virus persists in immunologically privileged sites and seeds into the circulation from infected cells such as the renal tubular epithelium. Due to a continuous endothelial cell layer and a thick basement membrane, these cells are, unlike hepatocytes, not readily accessible to the CTL. Their function as a viral reservoir has been demonstrated indirectly in the transgenic mice model (Ando et al, 1994a): intravascularly injected HBV-specific CTL were able to lyse only HBV-infected hepatocytes but not tissues like brain, kidney etc. that also expressed HBV antigen. When the CTL were injected directly into these tissues, i.e. beneath the kidney capsule or intracerebrally, however, they were also able to exert their cytopathic function. In humans it is also known that HBV replicates in extrahepatic tissues. Replicative forms of the virus have been detected in bile-duct epithelium and smooth-muscle cells (Blum et al, 1983), in pancreas, kidney and skin (Dejean et al, 1984), brain, endocrine tissues, lymph nodes (Yoffe et al, 1990; Beasley et al, 1993) and non-replicative forms in cells of the immune system themselves. Mitogenic stimulation of these cells induced viral replication (Korba et al, 1989). HBV might reach extrahepatic reservoirs where it cannot be eradicated by specific CTL. It is feasible that traces of virus may be sporadically released into the circulation from this putative reservoir, thereby maintaining the humoral and cellular immune response which prevents viral spread and protects the patient from re-infection and liver disease.

Hepatitis C

Why the hepatitis C virus is still not cleared as efficiently as the hepatitis B virus remains one of the obstacles of current research. Research has been hampered by the fact that most studies concentrate on patients with chronic infection only, since the acute stage of disease is most often clinically inapparent.

Unlike the situation in hepatitis B, in hepatitis C there are no antibody patterns that would allow a differentiation between different states or outcome of disease. So far, B cell epitopes have been identified within the hepatitis C virus envelope, core, NS3 and NS4 proteins (Cerino and Mondelli, 1991; Akatsuka et al, 1993; Ishida et al, 1993; Simmonds et al, 1993). Since most of the individuals develop persistent infection and 50% of them chronic hepatitis, the very existence of neutralizing antibodies has long been doubted. Recently, however, neutralizing antibodies have been detected in an in vitro system which uses continuous T cell lines for the replication of HCV (Shimizu et al, 1994). Accordingly, infectious plasma has been neutralized and used to passively immunize chimpanzees which were then protected from HCV infection in vivo (Shimizu et al, 1994). Vaccination of chimpanzees with recombinant envelope proteins expressed in mammalian cells also elicited high titres of neutralizing antibodies that protected from HCV challenge (Rosa et al, 1996). However, the situation is likely to be completely different in the infected patient—most B cell epitopes against which the antibodies are targeted are located within the hypervariable region HVR1 of the E2 envelope glycoprotein of HCV, and multiple sequences of this region have been identified in the same patient at any give time (Shimizu et al, 1994). Protective antibodies are therefore targeted against prior viral isolates which have already been replaced by mutated, new viral strains or by quasispecies in the infected patient; indeed, the data seem to support the hypothesis that the hepatitis C virus is able to 'escape' an efficient humoral immune response.

As far as the HLA class II-restricted T cell response to HCV is concerned, core, NS3 and NS4 proteins are most immunogenic. NS3, the putative helicase of the hepatitis C virus, is of special importance since a CD4$^+$ T cell response against this enzyme is found predominantly in patients who have recovered from acute viral hepatitis and therefore seems to be associated with viral clearance (Diepolder et al, 1995). In contrast to the class II-restricted immune response, the class I-restricted immune response of CD8$^+$ cells has not yet been studied in patients during or after recovery from acute hepatitis C.

CHRONIC HEPATITIS: VIRUS PERSISTENCE AND DISEASE PATHOGENESIS

Hepatitis B

Chronic hepatitis B is defined by the persistence of HBsAg and the absence of anti-HBs antibodies in the serum of infected patients in whom intrahepatic inflammatory activity can be histologically demonstrated for at least 6 months. The mechanisms that lead to persistence of the hepatitis B virus and development of chronic liver disease are not yet clear: to date, no specific characteristics of the HBV-specific immune response that would differentiate the 5% immunocompetent adults who develop chronic hepatitis from those who clear the infection have been identified. Specifically, there is no evidence for an association with certain HLA haplotypes.

As far as the virus is concerned, it has often been suggested that HBV mutants with amino acid changes in T cell, specifically CTL epitopes, might be able to evade the immune response of the host and induce chronic liver disease. However, some patients with acute hepatitis have been described who do not mount a CTL response against any of the published CTL epitopes (Rehermann et al, 1995b), but who are still able to clear the infection. Several authors have attributed this observation to an early, nonspecific immune response, such as NK cell activity (Nayersina et al, 1993; Rehermann et al, 1995b). In this respect, it is important to note that virus non-specific natural killer cells make up a fifth of all liver infiltrating cells during acute hepatitis, whereas they drop to below 10% in the chronic stage (Dienes et al, 1987).

Another important argument against viral escape from the immune response is the multispecificity of the CTL response which can be evaded only by a virus with mutations in most or all of the immunodominant epitopes (Bertoletti et al, 1991; Penna et al, 1992; Missale et al, 1993; Nayersina et al, 1993; Rehermann et al, 1995b,c). Some of the epitopes, however, are highly conserved between all viral subtypes. For example, the nucleocapsid epitope at amino acid position 141–151 is located in a functionally important domain because it overlaps a sequence (residues 145–156) at the carboxy terminus of the core protein that directs it to the nucleus (Eckhardt et al, 1991) and also plays a role in RNA encapsidation (Nassal, 1995). Within the viral envelope, epitopes HBsAg251–259 and HBsAg260–269 (Nayersina et al, 1993) are located within a viral sequence that is involved in transmembrane orientation of HBsAg and virus particle assembly (Eble et al, 1987). Finally, within the HBV polymerase protein, several epitopes are located within the reverse transcriptase and RNAse H domains (Rehermann et al, 1995b), regions that are essential for viral replication. Some of these epitopes are conserved even in the evolutionarily related retroviruses, emphasizing that these regions did not change for millions of years.

These results demonstrate that CTL can recognize highly conserved sequences that are essential in the viral life cycle and suggest that viral mutations at these sites which might otherwise allow the virus to escape from the immune response may not be compatible with survival of the virus.

Therefore, rather than viral escape from the immune response, alterations in the virus-specific immune response might be responsible for the development of persistent infections. Vertical transmission, i.e. from mother to child, accounts for most cases of chronic hepatitis B world-wide and in neonates persistent HBV infection is thought to be due to the induction of incomplete HBV-specific tolerance. Most neonates who develop persistent infection are born to HBsAg and HBeAg-positive mothers, and HBeAg is known to be able to cross the placental membrane. It has also been demonstrated within the umbilical cord of children of HBeAg-positive mothers (Arakawa et al, 1982; Lee et al, 1986). Within the thymus of the unborn child HBeAg would be recognized as self-antigen. The age of the child at the time point of infection is therefore crucial for the development of an HBV carrier state and correlates inversely with the rate of chronic infections (Beasley and Hwang, 1983).

The precise factors and mechanisms responsible for the varying forms of chronic inflammatory liver disease, and eventually irreversible liver injury resulting in cirrhosis and an increased risk of HCC, have been difficult to study since HBV has a limited host range, and tissue culture systems to propagate it do not exist. However, it is clear that the hepatitis B virus itself is not directly cytopathic (Chisari et al, 1989) and that the cellular immune response is involved in the pathogenesis of disease.

In this respect, it is important that a cellular infiltrate of the intrahepatic portal fields is characteristic for chronic hepatitis B and is thought to contribute to the development of piecemeal necrosis; these necroses are formed by dying hepatocytes and inflammatory infiltrates and reach from the portal fields into the liver parenchym. In addition to macrophages, histiocytes, fibroblasts and fibrocytes the majority of liver infiltrating cells are T lymphocytes: CD8$^+$ T cells are found in the space of Dissé in close contact with liver cells (Dienes et al, 1987) and the majority of these cells display activation markers, while most CD4$^+$ lymphocytes are found within the portal tracts and sinusoids (Eggink et al, 1982; Husby et al, 1982; Montano et al, 1983; Dienes et al, 1987). B cells are also present in the portal tracts and sinusoids where lymphoid follicles may form and act as peripheral lymphoid organs (Badardin and Desmet, 1984).

While the significance of liver-infiltrating lymphocytes could be studied only in a descriptive way using human liver biopsies, the development of an HBV-transgenic mouse model has made it possible to gain direct insight into intrahepatic pathogenetic mechanisms during HBV infection. Injection of HBV-specific CTL into transgenic mice expressing HBsAg on hepato-cytes revealed that the initiation of liver disease in acute hepatitis is based on antigen-specific recognition by CD8[+] lymphocytes which attach to HBsAg-positive hepatocytes and trigger them to undergo apoptosis (Ando et al, 1994b). Apoptotic hepatocytes appear as acidophilic Councilman bodies. During the first few hours after onset of acute hepatitis, CTL recruit antigen-non-specific inflammatory host cells, such as macrophages and NK cells, into the liver, creating an antigen-independent amplification cascade. This second step causes most of the histopathological manifestations of liver disease and can be prevented by neutralizing antibodies to gamma interferon (γIFN) or by inactivation of macrophages. Most commonly, however, hepatitis in this model is transient, non-fatal and does not result in chronic disease, presumably because the adoptively transferred CTL have a limited life span and cannot be replaced.

Hepatitis C

Unlike the situation in chronic HBV infection, the CTL response in chronic HCV infection is strong, polyclonal and multispecific, yet it is unable to clear the virus from the liver of patients with chronic hepatitis C.

As far as the class II-restricted T cell response is concerned, CD4[+] cells targeted against all viral proteins are detectable in the peripheral blood and the intrahepatic lymphocytic infiltrate in these patients. Specifically, the HCV core, NS3 and NS4 protein are recognized by most patients, and NS4-specific T cell clones have also been isolated from liver biopsies. Remarkably, a distinct clonotypic and functional difference was observed between peripheral blood and liver-derived NS4-specific T cells, suggest-ing a compartmentalization at the site of disease (Minutello et al, 1993).

Cytotoxic T cell epitopes have also been identified in all proteins of the hepatitis C virus. HCV-specific CD8[+] CTL with different HLA restrictions have been isolated from the blood and the liver of chronically infected patients (Koziel et al, 1992, 1993, 1995; Cerny et al, 1995) and chimpanzees (Erickson et al, 1993). Since antigen-non-specific stimulation is sufficient to expand HCV-specific CTL from liver biopsies, these cells must be present at fairly high frequency (Koziel et al, 1992, 1993, 1995). They are targeted against conserved as well as variable regions of the HCV proteins, so that the immune response can be described as polyclonal and multispecific as in acute hepatitis B. The differences in clearance of the hepatitis B and C viruses, however, suggest that distinct immunological and viral mechanims are responsible for the different courses of disease in both infections.

First, one factor to be considered is probably the relative antigenic load, which is high in chronic hepatitis B but low in hepatitis C. The weak peripheral blood T cell response in chronic hepatitis B could possibly be due to T cell exhaustion due to antigen overload, and it may contribute to viral persistence.

Second in hepatitis C, the quasispecies nature and the high mutation rate of the virus may contribute to an escape from the immune response. Evidence for this mechanisms is given by the report of the emergence of a CTL escape mutant in an HCV-infected chimpanzee (Weiner et al, 1995). In order to evaluate the potential mechanisms of viral persistence in HCV-infected patients, prospective analysis of viral nucleotide sequences in the context of the CTL response will be necessary.

Third, HCV may interfere with antigen processing or presentation by the hepatocyte, thereby diminishing its visibility to the immune system sufficiently to permit chronic low-grade inflammation to occur in the liver, but not enough for the immune response to kill all of the infected cells. The effect of co-expression of HCV proteins on the presentation of an independent antigen to the corresponding CTL will be needed to test this hypothesis.

Finally, it is also possible that the cytolytic function of the CTL is a bystander effect rather than the main antiviral effector function. In this respect, it is important to emphasize that CTL-derived cytokines, such as TNFα and γIFN can clear hepatocytes from the infecting hepatitis B virus without causing liver disease and that this effect is mediated by inhibition of viral gene expression and replication (Guidotti et al, 1994a,b, 1996). It is possible that the CTL produced in HCV infection do not secrete the appropriate cytokines or that the hepatitis C virus is less susceptible to them to permit viral clearance, but that the CTL are still capable of contributing to, or even causing, liver disease. If this pathway is required for viral clearance to be complete in an organ with as many potentially infected cells as the liver, viruses that are either intrinsically resistant to this pathway or that induce an immune response that does not produce the corresponding antiviral cytokines would have a survival advantage. It is possible that HCV falls into this category.

OUTLOOK: IMMUNOMODULATORY THERAPIES AS NEW STRATEGIES FOR CURING CHRONIC HEPATITIS

Although a vaccine to prevent HBV infection was derived from the plasma of chronic HBV carriers as early as 1980 (Szmuness et al, 1980) and is now readily available as recombinant major envelope (Valenzuela et al, 1982) or middle and major envelope proteins (Michel et al, 1984), there is still no causal cure for the millions of patients who are already chronically infected with the hepatitis B virus, and there is no vaccine at all to prevent hepatitis C virus infection. Since in most patients with chronic viral hepatitis, the virus has already gained access to many cells of the host, new vaccination strategies cannot rely on the induction of protective antibodies that complex viral particles and prevent them from infecting new host cell as previous vaccines did. New therapeutic approaches therefore aim at the induction of virus-specific cytotoxic T cell responses as an additional protective arm of the immune defence. The ability of CTL to both kill virus-infected host cells by induction of apoptosis and to cure them by release of specific cytokines is essential if the vaccinee is already chronically infected.

Three new therapeutic strategies which aim at the enhancement of the virus-specific cytotoxic T cell response of chronically infected patients should be described in detail. Because the role of a protective CTL response has first been established in HBV infection, these new therapeutic strategies have been designed predominantly for the treatment of patients with chronic hepatitis B.

The first evidence that vaccination of patients with chronic hepatitis could be successful came from a French study in which these patients were vaccinated with the conventional HBsAg vaccine (Pol, 1994). As a result, more patients than predicted in the natural course of disease were induced to synthesize HBV-specific protective antibodies, and were thus able to resolve the infection. While the immunological mechanisms of this vaccination strategy are still not clear, it is assumed that despite the huge excess of viral HBsAg in the peripheral blood of chronically infected patients, the administration of an additional small amount of exogenous HBsAg did manage to enhance a previously too-weak HBV-specific immune response (Celis et al, 1988; Jin et al, 1988; Penna et al, 1992). This effect could be due, for example, to an increased immunogenicity of the exogenous HBsAg because of its administration together with adjuvants or because of its route of administration, which could deliver it more directly to the regional lymph nodes and induce a specific HBV response. Most importantly, however, this study demonstrated that patients with chronic HBV infection do mount an HBV-specific immune response which can be enhanced by vaccination and thus lead to viral clearance and resolution of disease.

The identification of optimal CTL epitopes in the HBV envelope (Nayersina et al, 1993), nucleocapsid (Bertoletti et al, 1991) and polymerase (Rehermann et al, 1995b) proteins has therefore created the possibility to induce or enhance a CTL response directly by immunization with peptides containing the specific epitope sequence. On the basis of the results of animal studies which show that peptides alone are poor immunogens, but that administration of peptides in adjuvants (Tsai et al, 1992), liposomes (Guilhot et al, 1992) or direct attachment of lipids (Ferrari et al, 1990, 1991) enhances their immunogenicity, a lipopeptide-based vaccine has been developed in which an HLA-A2 restricted CTL epitope from HBV has been combined with a T helper epitope derived from tetanus toxoid and two molecules of palmitic acid and administered to HLA-A2-positive normal volunteers (Vitiello et al, 1995). In a phase I clinical trial, this vaccine induced HBV-specific CTL that killed autologous target cells which produced the corresponding HBV protein. These results raise the possibility that peptide-based vaccines might be used to induce HBV-specific HLA-class I-restricted memory CTL in patients with chronic hepatitis B virus infection. Studies to test this hypothesis are currently in progress.

Another new and very efficient vaccine strategy that was developed most recently is DNA-mediated immunization. Intramuscular administration of DNA expression vectors encoding sequences of the desired immunogenic protein under the control of an appropriate promoter has been shown to induce a strong immune response at the T and B cell level in mice (Davis et al, 1993) and to induce an anti-HBs response in otherwise tolerant HBsAg transgenic mice, which represents a model for the chronic HBV carrier state. Importantly, in these mice no liver injury was triggered despite the breaking of tolerance. If this vaccination strategy could eventually be applied to man it would have several advantages. First, DNA vectors are cheaper and easier to produce than antigenic proteins used in the current vaccines. Second, DNA immunization induces a strong CTL response as well as a T helper and antibody response to the expressed protein (Davis et al, 1993). These immune responses are not only directed against a multitude of viral epitopes, but also against naturally, i.e. endogenously processed epitopes. Indeed, in animals, DNA-mediated immunization has been shown to induce a CTL and antibody response against a broad variety of pathogens, such as influenza (Ulmer et al, 1993), HIV-1 (Wang et al, 1993a,b), rabies virus (Xiang et al, 1994) and, in recent unpublished studies in our laboratory, against the hepatitis B virus in normal mice and in HBV transgenic mice. Time will tell whether this promising new immunization strategy will prove to be effective enough to replace or to supplement the currently used vaccine.

If the concepts of hepatitis B immunobiology developed so far are correct, the strategy of boosting a virus-specific immune response in patients with chronic hepatitis by synthetic peptides, DNA-based or other vaccine strategies might tip the balance between virus and host, at least for HBV-infected patients. Whether the same strategies could be applied to chronic hepatitis C virus infection is still an open discussion because a protective role of an antiviral cytotoxic T cell response has not yet been sufficiently demonstrated. Clearly, more basic research on the specific virus–host interactions which determine the course of disease needs to be done, especially on those relatively rare individuals with acute HCV infection and on chronically infected patients who display sudden, severe disease flares and who completely eradicate the virus. Hopefully, these studies will allow us to gain a clearer picture of the role of the immune response in HCV clearance and disease pathogenesis so that a successful antiviral immunotherapy can be developed from which the more than 500 million people suffering from chronic viral hepatitis and its complications would benefit world-wide.

SUMMARY

More than 500 million people world-wide suffer from viral hepatitis which can be caused by a variety of distinct infectious agents. The spectrum of disease, which ranges from acute self-limited hepatitis to liver cirrhosis, not only reflects the different biological properties and pathogenicity of the hepatitis viruses, but is also the result of the specific interaction between each virus and the immune system of the infected host. The immune response plays a crucial role in the elimination of the infecting virus as well as in disease pathogenesis and is described in detail for acute and chronic hepatitis B and C virus infection. Acute hepatitis B virus infection is characterized by a vigorous, polyclonal cytotoxic T lymphocyte response against HBV that is not readily detectable in patients with chronic hepatitis B, suggesting that resolution of disease is mediated by the HBV-specific CTL response in these patients. Because traces of virus as well as HBV-specific CTL can perist for decades after clinical recovery, continuous priming of new CTL by minute traces of virus is thought to protect from re-activation of disease. In contrast, the hepatitis C virus causes chronic liver disease despite a polyclonal and multispecific immune response, suggesting that distinct immunological and viral mechanisms determine the different clinical outcome of HBV and HCV infection. Their implications for the development of immunomodulatory vaccines to cure patients with chronic viral hepatitis are discussed.

REFERENCES

Akatsuka T, Donets M, Scaglione L et al (1993)B cell epitopes on the hepatitis C virus nucleocapsid protein determined by human monospecific antibodies. *Hepatology* **18:** 503–510.

Alter MJ, Margolis HS, Krawczynski K et al (1992) The natural history of community-acquired hepatitis C in the United States. *New England Journal of Medicine* **327:** 1899–1905.

Ando K, Guidotti LG, Cerny A et al (1994a) Access to antigen restricts cytotoxic T lymphocyte function in vivo. *Journal of Immunology* **153:** 482–489.

Ando K, Guidotti LG, Wirth S et al (1994b) Class I restricted cytotoxic T lymphocytes are directly cytopathic for their target cells in vivo. *Journal of Immunology* **152:** 3245–3253.

Arakawa K, Tsuda F, Takahashi K et al (1982) Maternofetal transmission of IgG-bound hepatitis B e antigen. *Pediatric Research* **16:** 247–250.

Archer AC, Cohen BJ & Mortimer PP (1983) The value of screening blood donors for antibody to hepatitis B core antigen. *Journal of Clinical Pathology* **36:** 924–928.

Ashton-Rickardt PG & Murray K (1989) Mutants of the hepatitis B surface antigen that define some antigenically essential residues in the immunodominant a region. *Journal of Medical Virology* **29:** 196–203.

Badardin KA & Desmet VJ (1984) Interdigitating and dendritic reticulum cells in chronic active hepatitis. *Histopathology* **8:** 657–667.

Barnaba V, Franco A, Alberti A (1989) Recognition of hepatitis B envelope proteins by liver-infiltrating T lymphocytes in chronic HBV infection. *Journal of Immunology* **143:** 2650–2655.

Beasley RP & Hwang L (1983) Postnatal infectivity of hepatitis B surface antigen-carrier mothers *Journal of Infectious Diseases* **147:** 185–190.

Beasley RP, Hwang LY, Stevens CE et al (1993) Efficacy of hepatitis B immune globulin for prevention of perinatal transmission of the hepatitis B virus carrier state: final report of a randomized double-blind, placebo-controlled trial. *Hepatology* **3:** 135–141.

Bertoletti A, Ferrari C, Fiaccadori F, et al (1991) HLA class-I restricted human cytotoxic T cells recognize endogenously synthesized hepatitis B virus nucleocapsid antigen. *Proceedings of the National Academy of Sciences of the USA* **88:** 10 445–10 449.

Blum HE, Stowring L, Figus A et al (1983) Detection of hepatitis B virus DNA in hepatocytes, bile duct epithelium and, vascular elements by in situ hybridization. *Proceedings of the National Academy of Science of the USA* **80:** 6682–6685.

Brook MG, Karayiannis P & Thomas HC (1989) Which patients with chronic hepatitis B virus infection will respond to alpha-interferon therapy? A statistical analysis of predicitive factors. *Hepatology* **10:** 761–763.

Carmen WF, Zanetti AR, Karayiannis P et al (1990) Vaccine induced escape mutant of hepatitis B virus. *Lancet* **336:** 325–329.

Celis E, Ou D & Otvos L (1988) Recognition of hepatitis B surface antigen by human T lymphocytes. Proliferative and cytotoxic responses to a major antigenic determinant defined by synthetic peptides. *Journal of Immunology* **140:** 1808–1815.

Cerino A & Mondelli MU (1991) Identification of an immunodomonant B cell epitope on the hepatitis C virus non-structural region defined by human monoclonal antibodies. *Journal of Immunology* **147:** 2692–2696.

Cerny A, McHutchison JG, Pasquinelli C et al (1995) Cytotoxic T lymphocyte response to hepatitis C virus-derived peptides containing the HLA A2.1 binding motif. *Journal of Clinical Investigations* **95:** 521–530.

Chang LJ, Dienstag J, Ganem D & Varmus H (1989) Detection of antibodies against hepatitis B polymerase antigen in hepatitis ZB virus-infected patients. *Hepatology* **10:** 332–337.

Chisari FV, Ferrari C & Mondelli MU (1989) Hepatitis B virus structure and biology. *Microbiological Pathology* **6:** 311–325.

Choo Q-L, Kuo G, Weiner AJ et al (1989) Isolation of a cDNA clone derived from a blood-borne non-A, non-B viral hepatitis genome. *Science* **244:** 359–362.

Davis HL, Michel M-L & Whalen RG (1993) DNA-based immunization induces continuous secretion of hepatitis surface antigen and high levels of circulating antibody. *Human Molecular Genetics* **2:** 1847–1851.

Degos F, Lugassy C, Degott C et al (1988) Hepatitis B virus and hepatitis B-related viral infection in renal transplant recipients: a prospective study of 90 patients. *Gastroenterology* **94:** 151–156.

Dejean A, Lugassy C, Zafrani S et al (1984) Detection of hepatitis B virus DNA in pancreas, kidney and skin of two human carriers of the virus. *Journal of General Virology* **65:** 651–655.

Dienes HP, Hütteroth T, Hess G & Meuer SC (1987) Immunoelectron microscopic observations on the inflammatory infiltrates and HLA antigens in hepatitis B and non-A, non-B. *Hepatology* **7:** 1317–1325.

Diepolder HM, Zachoval R, Hoffmann RM et al (1995) Possible mechanism involving T lymphocyte response to non-structural protein 3 in viral clearance in acute hepatitis C virus infection. *Lancet* **346:** 1006–1007

Doherty PC, Allan W & Eichelberger M (1992) Roles of ab and gd T cell subsets in viral immunity. *Annual Review of Immunology* **10:** 123–151.

Eble BE, MacRae DR, Lingappa VR & Ganem D (1987) Multiple topogenic sequences determine the transmembrane orientation of hepatitis B surface antigen. *Molecular and Cellular Biology* **7:** 3591–3601.

Eckhardt SG, Milich DR & McLachlan A (1991) Hepatitis B virus core antigen has two nuclear localization sequences in the arginine-rich carboxyl terminus. *Journal of Virology* **65:** 575–582.

Eggink HF, Houthoff HJ, Huitema S et al (1982) Cellular and humoral immune reactions in chronic active liver disease. I. Lymphocyte subsets in liver biopsies of patients with untreated idiopathic autoimmune hepatitis, chronic active hepatitis B and primary biliary cirrhosis. *Clinical and Experimental Immunology* **50:** 17–24.

Erickson AL, Houghton M, Choo Q-L et al. (1993) Hepatitis C virus-specific CTL responses in the liver of chimpanzees with acute and chronic hepatitis C. *Journal of Immunology* **151:** 4189–4199.

Feitelson MA, Millman I, Duncan GD & Blumberg BS (1988) Presence of antibodies to the polymerase gene product(s) of hepatitis B and woodchuck hepatitis virus in natural and experimental infections. *Journal of Medical Virology* **24:** 121–126.

Ferrari C, Penna A, Bertoletti A et al (1990) Cellular immune response to hepatitis B virus-encoded antigens in acute and chronic hepatitis B virus infection. *Journal of Immunology* **145:** 3442–3449.

Ferrari C, Bertoletti A, Penna A et al (1991) Identification of immunodominant T cell epitopes of the hepatitis B virus nucleocapsid antigen. *Journal of Clinical Investigation* **88:** 214–222.

Franco A, Paroli M, Testa U et al (1992) Transferrin receptor mediates uptake and presentation of hepatitis B envelope antigen by T lymphocytes. *Journal of Experimental Medicine* **175:** 1195–1205.

Gilles PN, Fey G & Chisari FV (1992) Tumor necrosis factor-alpha negatively regulates hepatitis B virus gene expression in transgenic mice. *Journal of Virology* **66:** 3955–3960.

Guidotti LG, Ando K, Hobbs MV et al (1994a) Cytotoxic T lymphocytes inhibit hepatitis B virus gene expression by a noncytolytic mechanism in transgenic mice. *Proceedings of the National Academy of Sciences of the USA* **91**: 3764–3768.

Guidotti LG, Guilhot S & Chisari FV (1994b) Interleukin 2 and interferon alph/beta downregulate hepatitis B virus gene expression in vivo by tumor necrosis factor dependent and independent pathways. *Journal of Virology* **68**: 1265–1270.

Guidotti LG, Ishikawa T, Hobbs MV et al (1996) Intracellular inactivation of the hepatitis B virus by cytotoxic T lymphocytes. *Immunity* **4**: 35–36.

Guilhot S, Fowler P, Portillo G et al (1992) Hepatitis B virus (HBV) specific cytolytic T cell response in humans: production of target cells by stable expression of HBV-encoded proteins in immortalized human B cell lines. *Journal of Virology* **66**: 2670–2678.

Hadler SC, Judson FN, O'Mailley PM et al (1991) Outcome of hepatitis B virus infection in homosexual men and its relation to prior human immunodeficiency virus infection. *Journal of Infectious Diseases* **4**: 454–459.

Harrison TJ, Hopes EA, Oon CJ et al (1991) Independent emergence of a vaccine-induced escape mutant of hepatitis B virus. *Journal of Hepatology* **13**: S105–S107.

Hollinger FB (1990) Hepatitis B virus. In Fields BN, Knipe DM et al (eds) *Virology*, pp 2171–2236. New York: Raven Press.

Husby G, Blomhoff JP, Elgjo K & Williams SRC Jr (1982) Immunohistochemical characterization of hepatic tissue lymphocyte subpopulations in liver disease. *Scandinavian Journal of Gastroenterology* **17**: 855–860.

Ishida C, Matsumoto K, Fukada K et al (1993) Detection of antibodies to hepatitis C virus (HCV) structural proteins in anti-HCV-postive sera by an enzyme-linked immunosorbent assay using synthetic peptides as antigens. *Journal of Clinical Microbiology* **31**: 936–940.

Jin Y, Shih W-K & Berkower I (1988) Human T cell response to the surface antigen of hepatitis B virus (HBsAg). Endosomal and nonendosomal processing pathways are acessible to both endogenous and exogenous antigen. *Journal of Experimental Medicine* **168**: 293–306.

Korba BE, Cote PJ, Wells FV et al (1989) Natural history of woodchuck hepatitis virus infections during the course of experimental viral infection: molecular virologic features of the liver and lymphoid tissues. *Journal of Virology* **63**: 1360–1370.

Koziel MJ, Dudley D, Wong JT et al (1992) Intrahepatic cytotoxic T lymphocytes specific for hepatitis C virus in persons with chronic hepatitis. *Journal of Immunology* **149**: 3339–3344.

Koziel JM, Dudley D, Afdhal N et al (1993) Hepatitis C virus (HCV)-specific cytotoxic T lymphocytes recognize epitopes in the core and envelope proteins of HCV. *Journal of Virology* **67**: 7522–7532.

Koziel MJ, Dudley D, Afdhal N et al (1995) HLA class I-restricted cytotoxic T lymphocytes specific for hepatitis C virus. Identification of multiple epitopes and characterization of patterns of cytokine release. *Journal of Clinical Investigation* **96**: 2311–1221.

Krawczynski K & Bradley D W (1989) Enterically transmitted non-A, non-B hepatitis: identification of virus associated antigen in experimentelly infected cynomolgus macaques. *Journal of Infectious Diseases* **159**: 1042–1047.

Leary TP, Muerhoff AS, Simons JN et al (1996) Sequence and genomic organization of GBV-C: a novel member of the flaviviridae associated with human non-A-E hepatitis. *Journal of Medical Virology* **48**: 60–67.

Lee KSD, Lo KJ, Wu JC et al (1986) Prevention of maternal-infant hepatitis B virus transmission by immunization. The role of serum hepatitis B virus DNA. *Hepatology* **6**: 369–373.

Lemon SM, Whetter LE, Chang KH & Brown EA (1994) Recent advances in understanding the molecular virology of hepatoviruses: contrasts and comparisons with hepatitis C virus. In Nishioka K, Suzuki H, Mishiro S & Oda T (eds) *Viral Hepatitis and Liver Disease*, pp 22–27. Berlin: Springer-Verlag.

McDonald JA, Harris S, Water JA & Thomas HC (1987) Effect of human immunodeficiency virus (HIV) infection on chronic hepatitis B viral antigen display. *Journal of Hepatology* **4**: 337–342.

Michel M-L, Pontisso P, Sobczahk E et al (1984) Synthesis in animal cells of hepatitis B surface antigen particles carrying a receptor for polymerized human serum albumin. *Proceedings of the National Academy of Sciences of the USA* **81**: 7708–7712.

Minutello MA, Pileri P, Unutmaz D et al (1993) Compartmentalization of T-lymphocyte to the site of disease: intrahepatic CD4[+] T-cells specific for the protein NS4 of hepatitis C virus in patient with chronic hepatitis. *Journal of Experimental Medicine* **178**: 17–26.

Missale G, Redeker A, Person J et al (1993) HLA-A31 and Aw68 restricted cytotoxic T cell responses to a single hepatitis B virus nucleocapsid epitope during acute viral hepatitis. *Journal of Experimental Medicine* **177**: 751–762.

Montano L, Aranguibel F, Boffill M et al (1983) An analysis of the composition of the inflammatory infiltrate in autoimmune and hepatitis B virus-induced chronic liver disease. *Hepatology* **3**: 292–296.

Moretta L, Ciccone E, Mingari MC et al (1994) Human natural killer cells: origin, clonality, specificity, receptors. *Advances in Immunology* **55**: 341–358.

Nassal M (1995) The arginine-rich domain of the hepatitis B virus core protein is required for pregenome encapsidation and productive viral positive-strand DNA synthesis but not for virus assembly. *Journal of Virology* **66**: 4107–4116.

Nayersina R, Fowler P, Guilhot S et al (1993) HLA A2 restricted cytotoxic T lymphocyte responses to multiple hepatitis B surface antigen epitopes during hepatitis B virus infection. *Journal of Immunology* **150**: 4659–4671.

Nishihara T (1983) Intrahepatic distribution of T cell and T cell subsets in cases with type B chronic liver disease by peroxidase-labeled antibody method using monoclonal antibodies. *Gastroenterologia Japonica* **18**: 320–329.

Penna A, Fowler P, Bertoletti A et al (1992) Hepatitis B virus (HBV)-specific cytotoxic T-cell (CTL) response in humans: characterization of HLA class II-restricted CTLs that recognize endogenously synthesized HBV envelope antigens. *Journal of Virology* **66**: 1193–1198.

Pol S (1994) Specific vaccine therapy in chronic hepatitis B infection. *Lancet* **344**: 342.

Rehermann B, Ferrari C & Chisari FV (1995a) The cytotoxic T lymphocyte response persists long after recovery from acute viral hepatitis. *Hepatology* **22**: 223A (abstract).

Rehermann B, Fowler P, Sidney J et al (1995b) The cytotoxic T lymphocyte response to multiple hepatitis B virus polymerase epitopes during and after acute viral hepatitis. *Journal of Experimental Medicine* **181**: 1047–1058.

Rehermann B, Pasquinelli C, Mosier SM & Chisari FV (1995c) HBV sequence variation in CTL epitopes is not common in patients with chronic hepatitis B virus infection. *Journal of Clinical Investigation* **96**: 1527–1534.

Rehermann B, Lau D, Hoofnagle J & Chisari FV (1996) Cytotoxic T Lymphocyte responsiveness after resolution of chronic hepatitis B virus infection. *Journal of Clinical Investigation* **97**: 1–11.

Rosa D, Campagnoli S, Moretto C et al (1996) A quantitative test to estimate neutralizing antibodies to the hepatitis C virus: cytofluorimetric assessment of envelope glycoprotein 2 binding to target cells. *Proceedings of the National Academy of Sciences of the USA* **93**: 1759–1763.

Shimizu YK, Hijikita M, Iwamoto A et al (1994) Neutralizing antibodies against hepatitis C virus and the emergene of neutralization escape mutant viruses. *Journal of Virology* **68**: 1494–1500.

Simmonds P, Rose KA, Graham S et al (1993) Mapping of serotype-specific, immunodominatn epitopes in the NS4 region of hepatitis C virus (HCV): use of type-specific peptides to serologically differentiate infection with HCV type 1, 2 and 3. *Journal of Clinical Microbiology* **31**: 1493–1503.

Simons JN, Leary TP, Dawson GJ et al (1995) Isolation of novel virus-like sequences associated with human hepatitis. *Nature Medicine* **1**: 564–569.

Szmuness WA, Prince AM, Grady GF et al (1974) Hepatitis B infection: a point prevalence study in 15 U.S. hemodialysis center. *Journal of the American Medical Association* **227**: 901–906.

Szmuness W, Stevens CE, Harley EJ et al (1980) Hepatitis B vaccine: demonstration of efficacy in a controlled clinical trial in a high-risk population in the United States. *New England Journal of Medicine* **303**: 833–841.

Tam AW, Smith MJW, Guerra ME et al (1991) Hepatitis E virus (HEV): molecular cloning and sequencing of the full-length viral genome. *Virology* **185**: 120–131.

Tiollais P, Pourcel C & Dejean A (1985) The hepatitis B virus. *Nature* **317**: 489–495.

Tsai SL, Chen MY, Lai MY et al (1992) Acute exacerbations of chronic type B hepatitis are accompanied by increased T cell responses to hepatitis B core and e antigens. *Journal of Clinical Investigation* **89**: 87–96.

Ulmer JB, Donnelly JJ, Parker SE et al (1993) Heterologous protection against influenza by injection of DNA encoding a viral protein. *Science* **259**: 1745–1749.

Valenzuela P, Medina A, Rutter WJ et al (1982) Synthesis and assembly of hepatitis B virus surface antigen particles in yeast. *Nature* **298**: 347–350.

Vitetta ES, Fernandez-Botran R, Myers CD & Sanders VM (1989) Cellular interactions in the humoral immune response. *Advance in Immunology* **45**: 1–105.

Vitiello A, Ishioka G, Grey HM et al (1995) Development of a lipopeptide-based therapeutic vaccine to treat chronic HBV infection. 1. Induction of a primary cytotoxic T lymphocyte response in humans. *Journal of Clinical Investigation* **95:** 341–349.

Wands JR, Walker JR, Davis TT et al (1974) Hepatitis B in an oncology unit. *New England Journal of Medicine* **291:** 1371–1375.

Wang B, Boyer J, Srikantan V et al (1993a) DNA inoculation induces neutralizing immune responses against human immunodeficiency virus type 1 in mice and nonhuman primates. *DNA Cell Biology* **12:** 799–805.

Wang B, Ugen KE, Srikantan V et al (1993b) Gene inoculation generates immune responses against human immunodeficiency virus type 1. *Proceedings of the National Academy of Sciences of the USA* **980:** 4156–4160.

Waters JA, Kennedy M, Voet P et al (1992) Loss of the common 'a' determinant of hepatitis B surface antigen by a vaccine-induced escape mutant. *Journal of Clinical Investigation* **90:** 2543–2547.

Weimer T, Weimer K, Tu ZX et al (1989) Immunogenicity of human hepatitis B virus P-gene derived proteins. *Journal of Immunology* **143:** 3750–3759.

Weimer T, Schödel F, Jung M-C et al (1990) Antibodies to the RNase H domain of hepatatis B virus P protein are associated with ongoing viral replication. *Journal of Virology* **64:** 5665–5668.

Weiner A, Erickson AL, Kansopon J et al (1995) Persistent hepatitis C virus infection in a chimpanzee is associated with emergence of a cytotoxic T lymphocyte escape variant. *Proceedings of the National Academy of Sciences USA* **92:** 2755–2759.

Xiang ZQ, Spitalnick S, Tran M et al (1994) Vaccination with a plasmid vector carrying the rabies virus glycoprotein gene induces protective immunity against rabies virus. *Virology* **199:** 132–140.

Yoffe B, Burns DK, Bhatt HS & Combes B (1990) Extrahepatic hepatitis B virus DNA sequences in patients with acute hepatitis B infection. *Hepatology* **12:** 187–192.

Yuki N, Hayashi N, Kasahara A et al (1990) Detection of antibodies against the polymerase gene product in hepatitis B virus infection. *Hepatalogy* **12:** 193–198.

7

Cytochromes P450 and UDP-glucuronosyl-transferases as hepatocellular autoantigens

PETRA OBERMAYER-STRAUB
MICHAEL P. MANNS

Cytochromes P450 (P450) and UDP-glucuronosyltransferases (UGT) are drug metabolizing enzymes, which are known to be targets of auto-immunity. In this chapter general features of these two multigene families will be outlined. Hepatic diseases with autoimmune features will be described, where members of the cytochrome P450 and UGT protein families were identified to be targets of autoimmunity. Mechanisms involved in the formation of autoantibodies are discussed for drug induced hepatitis and factors that may be favourable for the induction of auto-immunity will be indicated in autoimmune hepatitis and virus associated autoimmunity. Autoimmune polyglandular syndrome type 1, a genetic disease with autoimmunity directed against various organs is especially interesting, since hepatic and several adrenal cytochromes P450 were shown to be autoantigens in organ specific autoimmunity.

THE SUPERGENE FAMILIES OF CYTOCHROMES P450 AND UDP-GLUCURONOSYLTRANSFERASES

Cytochromes P450 form a large superfamily of haem proteins with more than 150 genes (Nelson et al, 1993). In humans, cytochromes P450 fall into 13 families with members sharing a minimum of 40% sequence similarity. All cytochromes P450 are derived from a common ancestral gene (Nelson and Strobel, 1987). In man, cytochromes P450 are expressed in many organs, for example, skin, lung, adrenals, gonads, intestine, liver and kidney (Nebert and McKinnon, 1994). Some cytochrome P450 enzymes are essential in the biosynthetic pathways of steroids, prostaglandins and vitamin D3 (Nebert and McKinnon, 1994). Most of the cytochromes P450, however, are involved in drug metabolism. These enzymes belong to the cytochrome P450 families 1–4. Historically they are a result of plant–animal warfare. When animals started to adapt to terrestrial life, they had to feed on plants which had conquered the continents millions of years earlier. These plants had developed toxic substances, and animals adapted to this

Baillière's Clinical Gastroenterology —
Vol. 10, No. 3, September 1996
ISBN 0–7020–2187–3
0950–3528/96/030501 + 32 $12.00/00

source of nutrition by gene duplications of drug-metabolizing enzymes. Genes especially of the cytochrome P450 family 2 duplicated extensively, resulting in a huge number of different enzymes with broad and over-lapping substrate specificities (Nelson and Strobel, 1987). These enzymes are not only active in detoxification, but are also inducible by xenobiotics and drugs such as polycyclic-hydrocarbons and phenobarbital (Nebert and McKinnon, 1994). The most frequent reaction performed by cytochromes P450 is hydroxylation:

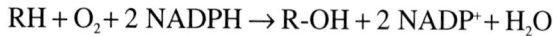

$$RH + O_2 + 2\ NADPH \rightarrow R\text{-}OH + 2\ NADP^+ + H_2O$$

Using four electrons from NADPH, cytochrome P450 reduces molecular oxygen to water and adds the second oxygen in the form of a hydroxyl group to the hydrophobic substrate (RH). This reaction represents the classical phase 1 of drug metabolism in which a given substrate is oxygenated, resulting in the 'functionalization' of the substrate (Figure 1). However, this reaction is not always beneficial (Figure 2). Sometimes the resulting product is unstable and reacts with cellular proteins or DNA. This process is called bioactivation. A well investigated example is paracetamol intoxication, which may result in hepatic failure (Thomsen et al, 1995). Activated reaction products may also be a cause of cancer by covalent modification of DNA. Adduct formation is also discussed as a mechanism for the induction of autoimmune reactions that are found with tienilic acid, dihydralazine and halothane (Beaune et al, 1993, 1994; van Pelt et al, 1995).

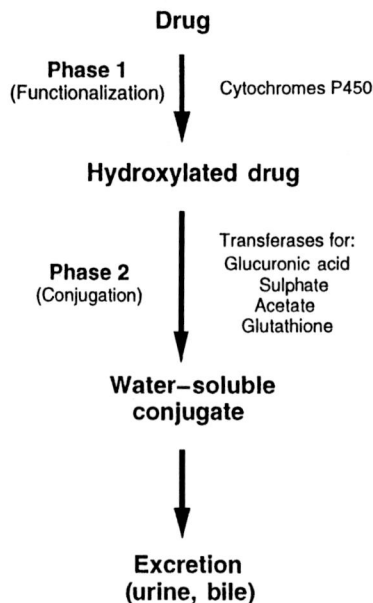

Figure 1. Phase 1 and phase 2 of drug metabolism.

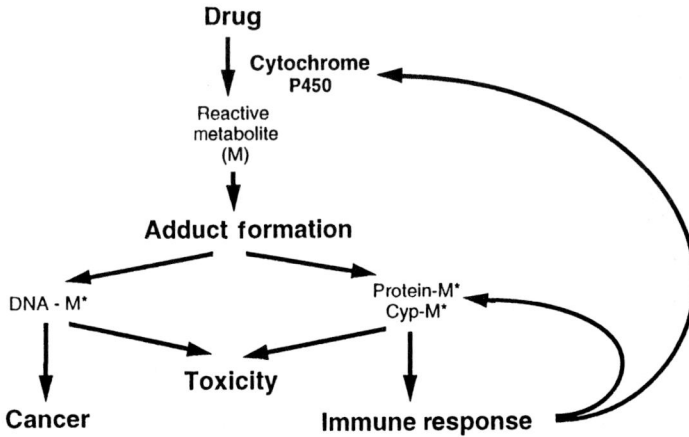

Figure 2. Bioactivation of drugs by cytochromes P450 and hypothesis for induction of autoimmunity in drug-induced hepatitis

Defects in drug-metabolizing cytochromes P450 under normal conditions will not result in disease or death. Therefore polymorphisms are found with a high frequency in the population (Gonzalez et al, 1988; Skoda et al, 1988). Defects in the structural genes or in regions responsible for splicing or regulation may lead to low-responder phenotypes. A well investigated example is the polymorphism of cytochrome P450 2D6 (Gonzalez et al, 1988). Cytochrome P450 2D6 is responsible for the metabolism of several classes of agent in man, including beta-blockers, anti-arrhythmic drugs and antidepressants (Nebert and McKinnon, 1994). Endogenous substrates are unknown. Up to 10% of the Caucasian population is deficient for drug metabolism mediated by cytochrome P450 2D6. Genetically this is due to at least eight different defective alleles that are found in the population (Nebert and McKinnon, 1994).

In phase 1 of drug metabolism, hydrophobic substances are hydroxylated by cytochromes P450. However, after hydroxylation the solubility in aqueous solutions is not increased enough for excretion. Therefore, chemicals with hydroxyl-, sulphydryl-, amino- or other polar groups are conjungated in a second reaction with hydrophilic substances, for example, glucuronic acid, sulphate, acetate or glutathione. These conjugation reactions together form phase 2 of drug metabolism (Figure 1). The most important reaction, the conjungation with glucuronic acid is performed by the UDP-glucuronosyltransferases (UGTs).

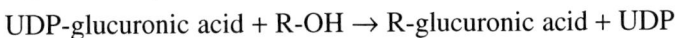

UDP-glucuronic acid + R-OH → R-glucuronic acid + UDP

UGT isoforms are found in liver, lung, intestine, gonads and brain (Burchell et al, 1994). As in hydroxylation, glucuronidation is performed by a multigene family. More than 16 human UGTs have been cloned, and the number of known human UGTs is steadily growing (Burchell et al,

1994). The most important endogenous substrate for glucuronidation is bilirubin, which is a major target for glucuronidation by UGT 1.1 (Burchell et al, 1994). Genetic defects severely impairing the activity of the bilirubin-GT result in Crigler Najjar syndrome type 1, which is characterized by unconjungated bilirubin levels of greater than 340 mM. As a result of the high bilirubin concentrations, infants often develop severe neurological damage from bilirubin encephalopathy (kernicterus). Less severe is Crigler Najjar type 2, which is characterized by bilirubin levels of 60–340 mM and can be treated by phenobarbital, which increases the levels of the bilirubin-transferase. Monoglucuronides in the bile are typical for patients with Crigler Najjar type 2 (Roy Chowdhury et al, 1989). A mild familial hyper-bilirubinaemia that affects about 5% of the population is Gilbert's syndrome, where the bilirubin levels are only moderately elevated (Fevery, 1981).

According to sequence homology, UGTs are subdivided in two families (Burchell et al, 1991, 1994). In humans, family 2 consists of more than nine known independent genes; in contrast, family 1 is encoded in a large gene cluster (Ritter et al, 1992) (Figure 3). Each gene consists of five

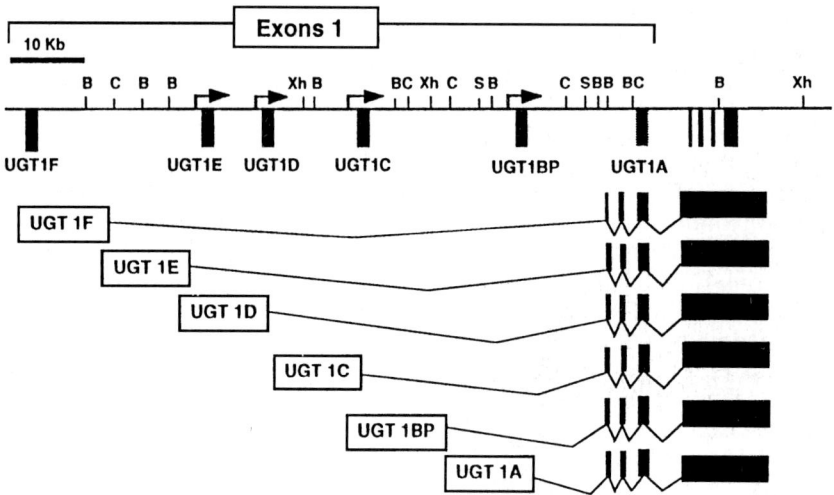

Figure 3. Gene locus for family 1 UDP-glucuronosyltransferases according to Ritter et al (1992).

exons, exons 2 to 5 being the same for all family 1 UGTs (Figure 4). In contrast, at least 11 independently regulated exons 1 are present; these are linked to the constant exons 2–5 by differential splicing. Therefore, mutations in the constant exons apply to the whole family 1 UGTs (Ritter et al, 1992).

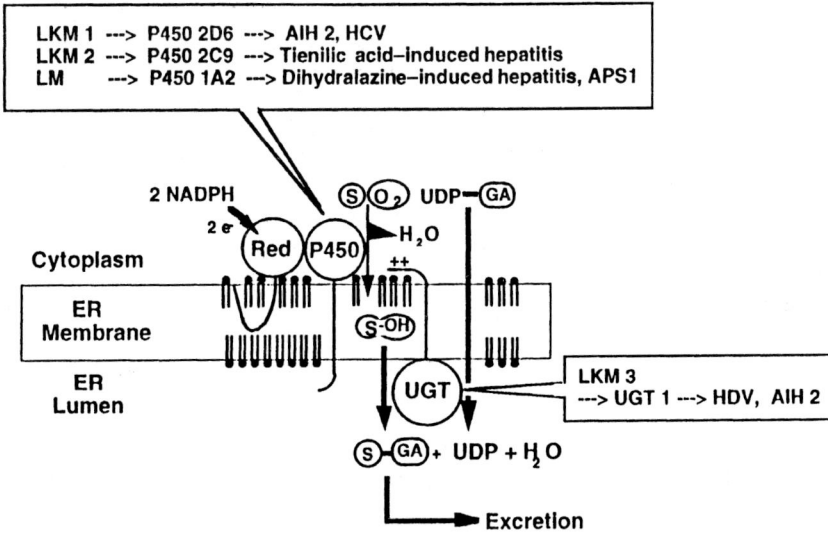

Figure 4. Cytochromes P450 and UDP-glucuronosyltransferases are autoantigens in different liver diseases. Modified according to Iyanagi et al (1986).

MULTIPLE PATHOGENIC PROCESSES LEAD TO THE DEVELOPMENT OF CHRONIC HEPATITIS

Investigations concerning the aetiology and pathogenesis of chronic hepatitis are subject to rapid progress. Today, chronic hepatitis is classified in several subgroups according to the aetiology of the disease (Table 1). Most cases of chronic hepatitis are due to an infection with hepatitis viruses B, C and D. A recently discovered virus, hepatitis G, has just entered discussion. The diagnosis of viral hepatitis is based on the presence of antibodies directed against viral proteins or on the detection of the viral nucleic acids by PCR. Some of the patients infected with hepatitis C or D also develop autoimmune reactions, resulting in the production of auto-antibodies. This phenomenon is called 'virus-induced autoimmunity'. A second group of patients with chronic hepatitis suffers from autoimmune hepatitis (AIH). Virus markers are absent; however, various autoantibodies exist. According to the organelle where the autoantigen comes from, autoimmune hepatitis is subdivided into three different subtypes. AIH type 1 is characterized by anti-nuclear autoantibodies, and AIH type 2 by microsomal antibodies specific for liver and kidney (LKM) or for liver alone (LM) (Bourdi et al, 1990; Manns et al, 1991). AIH type 3 is characterized by autoantigens directed against cytokeratins 8 and 18 (SLA) (Manns, 1991). In about 10% of cases of chronic hepatitis markers of infection with a known virus are absent and autoantibodies are missing. These ill-defined cases of chronic hepatitis represent a group of diseases of presumably mixed yet unknown aetiology, and they are therefore categorized as 'cryptogenic hepatitis'. A small group of patients with chronic hepatitis suffer from immunoallergic reactions after treatment with specific drugs. The disease of patients in this group is called 'drug-induced hepatitis' and is also characterized by autoantibodies.

In all cases of chronic hepatitis the immune system plays a major role. Some hepatotropic viruses are well adapted to evade elimination by the immune system, for example, most of the infections with hepatitis C become chronic (Dienstag, 1990). However, some immune defence mechanisms still work. Viral antigens that are expressed in the hepatocytes are presented to the immune system via MHC molecules, and viral surface molecules may be targets for detection by specific antibodies and the complement system. Therefore, lymphocytic infiltrates are found in the infected liver tissue. The chronic immune attack causes continuous liver cell damage, as measured by elevated levels of transaminases. Continuous cell lysis and stimulation of immune cells may be a factor contributing to the formation of autoantibodies that are frequently detected with hepatitis C and D. However, the rather high prevalence of autoantibodies in hepatitis C and D, compared to their absence in hepatitis A and B, indicates specific mechanisms, for example, cross-reaction of viral antigens with native hepatic antigens at the level of sequence similarity or by mimicking tertiary structures.

In autoimmune hepatitis the immune system attacks the liver tissue in the absence of viral infection. Lymphocytic infiltrates are present, leading to severe cell damage and cirrhosis. In contrast to viral hepatitis, the immune response in AIH is focused on self-antigens. This condition can be treated by immunosuppression, which is of great benefit for patients suffering from AIH. A good model for studying the development of autoimmune reactions and their underlying defects in the immune response is the autoimmune

Table 1. Diagnostic criteria for autoimmune hepatitis.

Diagnostic criteria	Score
Hypergammaglobulinaemia	+3
Autoantibodies	
ANA, SMA, LKM1	+3
SLA, ASGPR, LP	+2
AMA	−2
Female sex	+2
AST/ALT <3.0	+2
Complete response to immunosuppression	+2
Virus markers	
Anti-HAV IgM, HBsAg, anti-HBc IgM	−3
HCV RNA (PCR)	−3
Anti-HCV	−2
Other virus infections	−3
Ethanol intake	
Males <35 g/day females <25 g/day	+2
Immunogenetics: HLA-B8-Dr3 or DR4	+1

polyglandular syndrome type 1 (APS1), a rare genetic disease that is due to a defect in a single gene locus (Aaltonen et al, 1994). APS1 patients suffer from candidiasis and autoimmune reactions directed against various organs, for example, parathyroiditis, adrenals, ovaries, liver and skin (Ahonen et al, 1990). New disease components develop throughout life, the average patients suffering from five to six of them. About 20% of patients affected by APS1 will develop hepatitis (Ahonen et al, 1990). Therefore a continuous monitoring of the reactivity of B- and T-cells to tissue-specific autoantigens may help us to gain further insights into the genetically determined multi-antigen autoimmune disease.

In patients treated with certain drugs, drug-induced hepatitis is found with a low frequency. It is necessary to distinguish the direct toxic effect of drugs, which occurs during the period of drug treatment in a dose-dependent manner from the immunoallergic reaction that is called drug-induced hepatitis. In contrast, immune allergic responses occur after a latent period only in few patients, and they are dependent on the immune system. In drug-induced hepatitis adducts between a reactive metabolite of the drug and cellular problems stimulate an immune response. This immune response is directed against self-proteins, mostly the enzyme that performed the metabolic activation of the drug. This effect leads to mild toxicity in all patients. However, in a few patients treated with the drug the immune system will start reacting against drug adducts and the native forms of the target proteins. This reaction will manifest as drug-induced hepatitis that is characterized by severe liver damage. As only small numbers of patients suffer from these immunoallergic reactions, it is likely that immunological and metabolic aberrations in these patients may be involved in the development of drug induced-hepatitis.

As shown in Table 2, LKM autoantibodies are detected in many types of chronic hepatitis. The LKM autoantibodies are well characterized, and numerous autoantigens were identified at the molecular level. Most of the known antigens belong to the group of drug-metabolizing enzymes, cytochromes P450 and UGTs. In spite of a high degree of sequence similarity between the different cytochromes P450, the autoantibodies are specific for single members of the cytochrome P450 family or for a distinct UGT sequence. Autoantibodies directed against different targets are detected with the different types of chronic hepatitis (Figure 4). In the following chapters potential processes leading to the formation of LKM autoantibodies in drug-induced hepatitis will be presented, and the identity and clinical relevance of LKM autoantibodies in autoimmune and virus-induced hepatitis will be discussed.

DRUG-INDUCED HEPATITIS

Because of the central role of the liver in xenobiotic metabolism, this organ is also an important target for adverse drug reactions. Hydroxylation by cytochromes P450 may lead to the formation of unstable metabolites that bind to cellular proteins or DNA. This direct toxic effect may lead to cell

Table 2. Antibodies as diagnostic markers in chronic hepatitis.

Hepatitis type	HBsAg	HBV-DNA	Anti-HDV (HDV-RNA)	Anti-HCV (HCV-RNA)	ANA	LKM/LM	SLA/LP
B	+	+/-	-	-	-	-	-
C	-	-	-	+	+/-	2% P450 2D6	-
D	+	-	+	-	-	59 kDa, 70 kDa 10% UGT1	-
Autoimmune hepatitis							
Type 1	-	-	-	-	+	-	-
Type 2	-	-	-	-	+/-	P450 2D6, 64 kDa	-
Type 3	-	-	-	-	+/-	-	+
Autoimmune hepatitis in APS-1	-	-	-	-	+/-	P450 1A2 LKM[a]	-
Drug-induced hepatitis	-	-	-	-	+/-	P450 1A2, P450 2C9, LKM[b]	-
Cryptogenic hepatitis	-	-	-	-	-	-	-

[a] Target is not identified yet.
[b] See Table 1.

death or cancer (Guengerich, 1993). If the protein adducts formed in this process are presented to the immune system as neoantigens, this process may eventually lead to an immune response, including the production of autoantibodies, inflammation and necrosis (Figure. 5). Potential mechanisms responsible for this indirect type of toxicity are discussed for hepatitis induced by tienilic acid, by dihydralazine and by halothane.

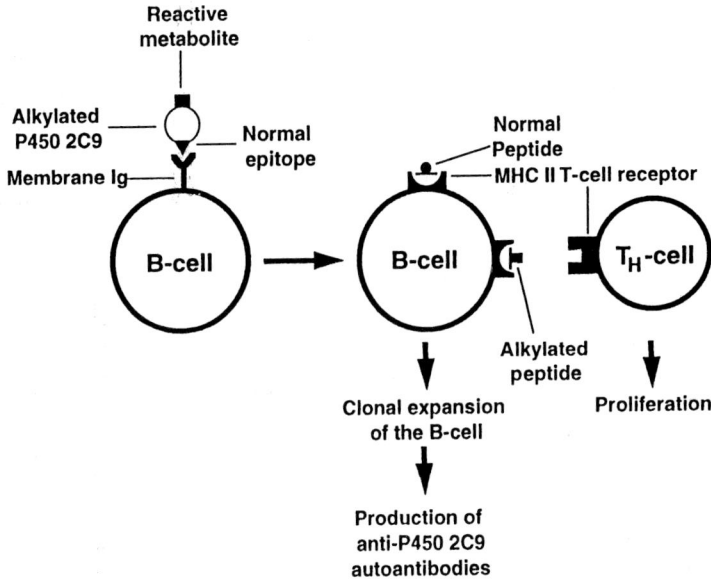

Figure 5. A hypothetical mechanism for the generation of the LKM2 autoantibody (anti-P450 2D6). Modified according to Pessayre (1993).

Tienilic acid-induced hepatitis

Tienilic acid is an uricosuric drug used in the treatment of hypertension (Figure 6A). It was withdrawn from the market a few years after introduction because of clinical reports of rare, but severe, hepatotoxicity (Zimmerman et al, 1984). During treatment, an asymptomatic increase of transaminases was detected in 7% of the patients. However, in 0.1–0.7% of patients, clinical hepatitis developed (Zimmerman et al, 1984). Female and male patients were affected equally, and liver damage was found to be dose-independent. The reaction always occured with significant delay, the onset of hepatitis being observed after 14–240 days of drug treatment. Liver biopsies from 27 patients revealed acute hepatitis in 20 cases, with centrilobular necrosis in 15 and spotty panlobular injury in five patients (Zimmerman et al, 1984). The livers were infiltrated by neutrophils, eosinophils and lymphocytes. After discontinuation of drug treatment the liver damage resolved. Rechallenge with the drug resulted in the recurrence of symptoms in 95% of patients—but after a shorter time period than before

A   Tienilic acid

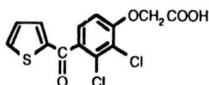

B   Reactions of the activated metabolites of tienilic acid

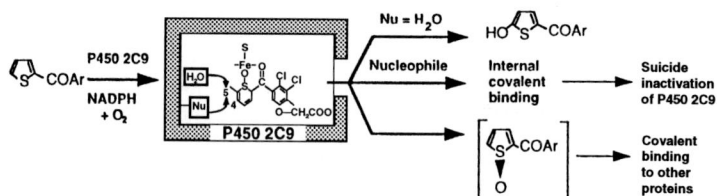

Figure 6. (A) Chemical structure of tienilic acid. (B) Reactions of the activated metabolites of tienilic acid. According to Beaune et al (1994).

(Zimmerman et al, 1984). One patient was reported to have suffered four sucessive episodes with progressive shortening of the time interval between the onset of tienilic acid administration and the onset of hepatitis (3 months, 12 days, 3 days and 6 hours) (Bernuau et al, 1981).

A specific antibody, directed against unmodified liver and kidney microsomal proteins, was detected in 60% of patients suffering from hepatitis after administration of tienilic acid; this antibody is not present in sera from healthy controls (Homberg et al, 1984, 1985). This specific autoantibody was called anti-liver-kidney microsomes type 2 (LKM2). The target of this autoantibody cross-reacts with rat P450 2C11. When tested against several human cytochromes P450 expressed in yeast—including P450 1A1, P450 1A2, P450 2C9 and P450 2C18—anti-LKM2 sera reacted specifically with cytochrome P450 2C9, the most abundant cytochrome P450 in the human liver and the major tienilic acid metabolizing enzyme (Lopez-Garcia et al, 1993; Lecoeur et al, 1994).

Based on the available data, a mechanism for LKM2 induction in patients with tienilic acid-induced hepatitis was proposed (Figure 6B) (Beaune et al, 1994). According to this hypothesis, tienilic acid is activated in the active centre of P450 2C9 to form a reactive sulphoxide. This sulphoxide covalently binds to the metabolizing enzyme, cytochrome P450 2C9, and causes enzyme inactivation. Some molecules leave the active centre and bind to other liver proteins or to glutathione. As most sulphoxides will be eliminated by glutathione in the hepatocyte, cytochrome P450 2C9 is the main target protein of activated tienilic acid metabolites (Lopez-Garcia et al, 1993). Hence, no autoantibodies directed against other hepatic proteins are found. After suicide inactivation, cytochrome P450 2C9 may be presented to the immune system and cause a circumvention of T cell tolerance by a mechanism that was proposed by

Pessayre (Figure 5) (Pessayre, 1993). The basis of this hypothesis is the fact that quiescent autoreactive B-lymphocytes were demonstrated to be present at low levels in humans. After mild liver injury, of the type found in many patients after drug application, such a quiescent autoreactive B-lymphocyte may bind cytochrome P450 2C9. The protein is internalized and processed into small peptides that bind to molecules of HLA class II in a specialized compartment of the B-cells. In the form of small peptides, alkylated and native peptides will be presented on the surface of the B-cell. While T-cells recognizing self-peptides are usually not present, T-helper cells recognizing the alkylated 'modified-self' peptides might be present in the population. After presentation of the modified-self peptide to T-helper cells, both B- and T-cells are activated by the bidirectional signalling and start proliferating. At the B-cell level, this event results in clonal expansion, maturation and production of autoantibodies directed against a normal unmodified domain of cytochrome P450 2C9, the LKM2 autoantibody. However, it is not yet known whether this LKM2 autoantibody is just a side-product of the pathogenic process or whether this autoantibody is directly involved in liver cell injury. A direct impact of the LKM2 autoantibody on hepatic injury would require the LKM2 autoantibody to bind directly to the hepatocytes and activate cytotoxic T-cells and the complement system.

A prerequisite for such a pathogenic role would be the presence of cytochrome P450 2C9 on the surface of the hepatocytes (Beaune et al, 1994). This topic, however, has been controversally discussed for many years. Several groups failed to detect cytochromes P450 in the plasma membrane of hepatocytes (De Lemos-Chiarandini et al, 1987a,b; Trautwein et al, 1993, Yamamoto et al, 1993a). However, others described the presence of several cytochromes P450 in the hepatic plasma membrane (Jarasch et al, 1979; Staciecki and Oesch, 1980; Lenzi et al, 1984; Loeper et al, 1990, 1993; Wu and Cederbaum, 1992; Robin et al, 1995). Loeper isolated rat and human hepatocytes and prepared the plasma membrane fraction. Indirect immunofluorescence, immuno-electron microscopy and Western blotting with highly enriched plasma membrane fractions revealed the presence of cytochromes P450 on the surface of the hepatocytes. The cytochromes P450 in the plasma membrane fraction also were shown to be enzymatically active. However, doubt about the surface expression persisted, and Robin reinvestigated the topic of surface expression of cytochromes P450 on the basis of P450 2B1, using cultivated rat hepatocytes before and after induction with phenobarbital (Robin et al, 1995). Using FACs analysis and electron microscopy, the authors demonstrated the surface expression of cytochromes P450 2B and were able to demonstrate that the cytochromes P450 2B follow a vesicular route from the ER to the Golgi apparatus. Interestingly they found that cytochrome P450 2B, which is usually expressed on the cytoplasmic surface of the ER, is located at the outer surface of the plasma membrane (Robin et al, 1995). A surface location of cytochromes P450 would suggest a pathogenic role of autoantibodies in tienilic acid-induced hepatitis. However, in addition to potential antibody-related processes, other disease mechanisms have to be involved because a significant proportion of patients with tienilic acid-induced hepatitis are void of detectable autoantibodies (Homberg et al, 1984, 1985).

Dihydralazine-induced hepatitis

After chronic treatment with the hypertensive drug dihydralazine, a large number of patients with hepatitis were reported (Stricker, 1992). This type of drug-induced hepatitis affected more female than male patients, with a female:male ratio of 2.7 (Roschlau, 1986). Most patients were of the slow acetylator phenotype (Siegmund et al, 1985). The onset of hepatitis was usually delayed, with a latent period of several months, and it resolved after the discontinuation of the treatment (Roschlau, 1986). Rechallenge with the drug resulted in recurrence of hepatitis, usually but not always after a shorter time interval (Reinhardt et al, 1985). Histology showed lesions of acute or subacute hepatitis with centrilobular necrosis, often associated with bridging necrosis. The inflammatory infiltrate included mononuclear cells, neutrophils and eosinophils (Roschlau, 1983). In 18 patients a positive lymphocyte transformation was reported (Kunze et al, 1985).

Dihydralazine hepatitis is associated with liver microsomal antibodies (LM) that do not stain kidney sections (Homberg et al, 1984; Nataf et al, 1986; Boccaccio et al, 1987; Bourdi et al, 1990). The LM autoantibody recognizes a single band in human liver microsomes that was detected by all LM sera tested. However, a high variability in the titre of the auto-antibody was observed (Bourdi et al, 1990). Using purified preparations of human cytochromes P450, the target protein was identified as cytochrome P450 1A2 (Bourdi et al, 1990). LM autoantibodies are very specific. Despite a high sequence homology between cytochromes P450 1A1 and P450 1A2, no cross-reaction with cloned human P450 1A1 is observed (Bourdi et al, 1992). LM autoantibodies react with slices of rat liver tissue and dot blots of purified rat cytochrome P450 1A2. In contrast, they are unable to react to rat antigens in Western blots, indicating that confor-mation-specific epitopes on the native protein are recognized (Bourdi et al, 1990).

For the development of LM autoantibodies, Beaune and his colleagues proposed a mechanism that is based on the metabolites detected in human plasma and urine and on evidence that cytochrome P450 1A2 acts as the dihydralazine-activating enzyme (Figures 7 and 8) (Schröder et al, 1986; Beaune et al, 1994).

Several pathways of metabolization were proposed for the turnover of dihydralazine; however, two pathways seem to be important (Schröder et al, 1986). One pathway, which is believed to result in detoxification, is dependent on the activity of the N-acetyltransferase. The product is an acetyl conjungate (Bock, 1992). A second oxidative pathway was shown to contribute to the metabolic activation of dihydralazine, forming electrophilic reaction intermediates. Indirect evidence suggests that cytochrome P450 1A2 is the major enzyme active in this oxidative pathway, resulting in adduct formation and the production of 'neoantigens' (Beaune et al, 1994; Bourdi et al, 1994). As a result, the equilibrium

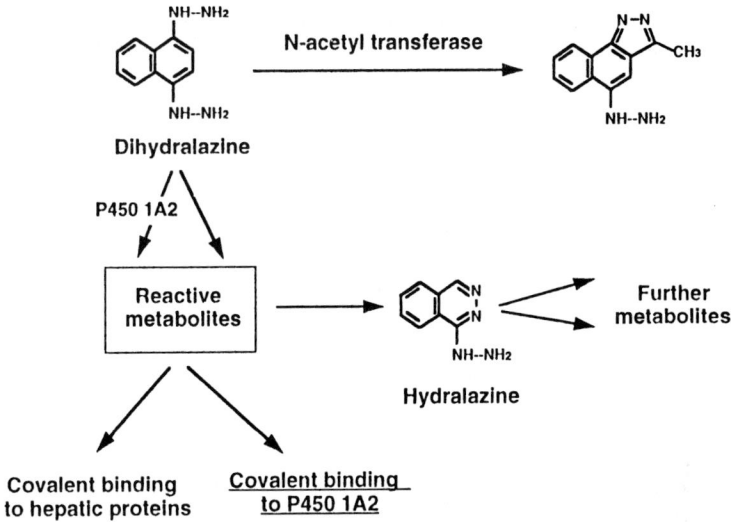

Figure 7. Potential detoxification and bio-activation pathways of dihydralazine. Modified according to Beaune et al (1994).

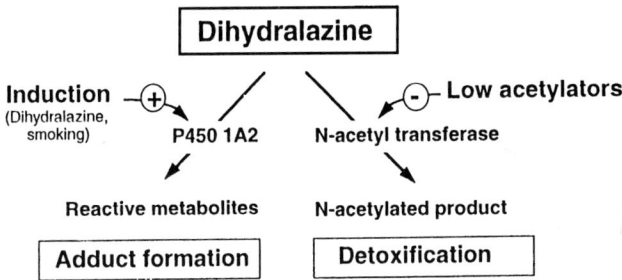

Figure 8. Factors modulating the balance between bio-activation and detoxification of dihydralazine. According to Beaune et al (1994).

between acetylation and bio-activation may be critical for the development of the disease. This equilibrium may be influenced by environmental and genetic factors. Induction of cytochrome P450 1A2 by dihydralazine was demonstrated in human hepatocytes, suggesting that, with prolonged administration of this hypertensive drug, the oxidative metabolism and the production of neoantigens may increase (Bourdi et al, 1992). Cytochrome P450 1A2 is further subject to induction by smoking (Beaune et al, 1994), suggesting that smokers should be over-represented in patients with dihydralazine hepatitis if the hypothesis presented in Figures 7 and 8 is correct. Unfortunately, the smoking status of patients with dihydralazine hepatitis has not yet been investigated. Finally, the absence of *N*-acetyl-transferase activity in people with the slow acetylator phenotype—50% of the Caucasian population—may increase adduct formation and cause the over-representation of slow acetylators in patients with dihydralazine hepatitis.

Halothane-induced hepatitis

In 1956 halothane was introduced as an anaesthetic agent and has been widely used since then. Two types of hepatitis are known that may be produced by halothane. In about 20% of recipients a mild, asymptomatic increase of serum transaminases occurs (Trowel et al, 1975; Wright et al, 1975). This mild disease may be directly caused by a toxic mechanism of halothane, since, in 7/7 patients anaesthetized with halothane, mild ultra-structural lesions were detected (Sindelar et al, 1982). In about 1/10 000 patients anaesthetized for the first time with halothane severe hepatitis, termed 'halothane hepatitis', will develop. Halothane hepatitis is character-ized by severe liver failure and extensive, predominantly centrilobular, liver cell necrosis. Fulminant hepatitis with hepatic encephalopathy frequently develops and is associated with a high rate of fatality (Zimmerman, 1978). Multiple exposure to halothane increases the susceptibility to halothane hepatitis and the severity of liver damage increases with shortening of the interval between the anaesthesia. The latent period of jaundice is 12 days after single exposure, 7 days after the second and 5 days after the third exposure (Zimmerman, 1978). Female, obese and late middle-age people are at an increased risk of developing this type of hepatitis (Zimmerman 1978; Ray and Drummond, 1991). Indications for a genetic component were found in three pairs of closely related women (Eade et al, 1981). Metabolic aberrations may contribute to the development of halothane hepatitis because, in patients with halothane hepatitis and about 50% of their family members, an enhanced sensitivity towards electrophilic metabolites of phenytoin was found. Hypersensitivity manifestations are frequently observed, including fever, eosinophilia, rash, elevated levels of circulating immune complexes and a variety of circulat-ing autoantibodies (Walton et al, 1976; Homberg et al, 1985). Inflammatory infiltrates of the liver contain mononuclear cells, neutrophils and some-times eosinophils (Zimmerman, 1978). Thymidine incorporation assays revealed lymphocyte stimulation in the presence of halothane in 10/15 patients with halothane hepatitis, which was not detectable in healthy controls or in patients exposed to halothane without subsequent liver damage (Paronetto and Popper, 1970).

Halothane is metabolized by cytochromes P450 to a variety of reactive metabolites that bind to hepatic macromolecules (Kenna et al, 1990a; Kenna and van Pelt, 1994). Two metabolic pathways—a reductive and an oxidative pathway—have been described (Figure 9) (Sipes et al, 1980). The reductive metabolism is discussed as the cause of the mild-form liver injury that results from direct toxicity of halothane and leads to the formation of a free radical that, in turn, triggers lipid peroxidation (Plummer et al, 1982; Knights et al, 1988; Kenna and van Pelt, 1994). The oxidative pathway predominates in humans. It leads to the formation of the highly reactive trifluoroacetylchloride (CF₃COCl) (Sipes et al, 1980). This reactive metabolite may react with water to form trifluoroacetate, bind to the lysine residues of proteins or bind to phospholipids (Figure 9) (Trudell et al, 1991; Kenna and van Pelt, 1994). Studies using rat microsomes after induction with various enzyme-inducing agents, and studies using purified cytochrome P450, suggest that cytochrome P450 2E1 might be involved in the oxidative metabolism of halothane (Gruenke et al, 1988; Kenna et al, 1990b; Koop, 1992). A number of soluble rat hepatic microsomal proteins were shown to be trifluoroacetylated (Table 3). It was suggested that, in these soluble ER-proteins, the KDEL motif that prevents these proteins from migrating to the Golgi apparatus is trifluoroacetylated by halothane (Pumford et al, 1993). Therefore these proteins might be excreted, taken up by Kupfer cells, processed into peptides and trigger the immunization process. Trifluoroacetylated proteins of unknown identity are also

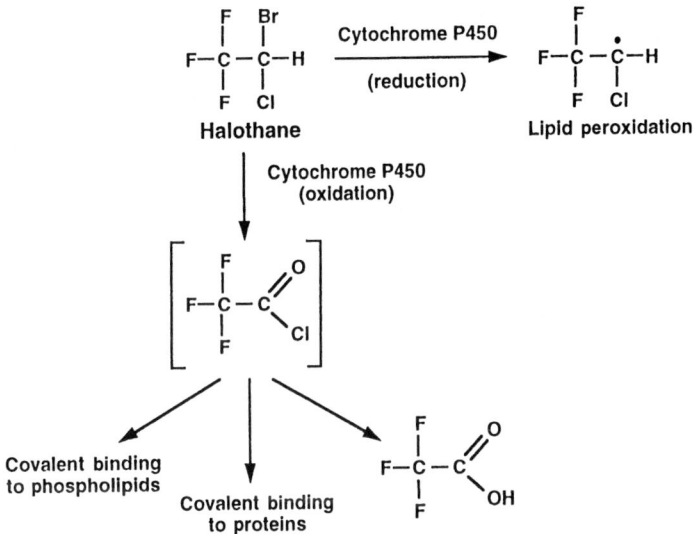

Figure 9. Metabolism of halothane.

Table 3. Hepatic trifluoroacetylated antigens recognized by patient sera with halothane hepatitis.

Molecular weight	Protein
54 kDa	Cytochrome P450?
57 kDa	Protein disulphide isomerase
58 kDa	?
59 kDa	Microsomal carboxylesterase
63 kDa	Calreticulin
80 kDa	ERp72
82 kDa	BiP/GRP78
100 kDa	ERp99

detectable on the membrane of the hepatocyte, where they might be a target for the immune system even as the described endoplasmic proteins.

Further work suggests in addition to antibodies directed against trifluoro-acetylated proteins, antibodies directed against conformational epitopes on native proteins also exist. These autoantibodies can be detected with indirect immunofluorescence in 25% of sera from patients with halothane hepatitis. They are directed against microsomal proteins of the liver and kidney (LKM). Using those native proteins of the targets of trifluoro-acetylation which have been identified, little if any activity is found in Western blots. If, however, the native proteins are used in ELISA, a significant proportion of the sera also recognizes the native proteins, demonstrating that many autoantibodies are directed against confor-mational epitopes of these proteins (Pohl et al, 1991; Butler et al, 1992; Pumford et al, 1993; Smith et al, 1993). Further autoantibodies directed against variable normal liver proteins also occur.

In spite of the multiplicity of neoantigens induced by halothane, the development of halothane hepatitis is a rather rare event. A possible explanation for the low frequency of immunoallergic reactions due to halothane may be that molecular mimicry provides tolerance against the trifluoroacetylated lysine domains (Gut et al, 1992, 1993). This hypothesis is based on the finding that monospecific rabbit antibodies directed against the N_e-trifluoroacetyl-lysine-domain specifically recognize two unmodified hepatic protein in Western blots with molecular weights of 52 kDa and 74 kDa. The 74 kDa protein was identified as the dihydrolipoamide acetyl transferase (E2) subunit of pyruvate dehydrogenase complex (Christen et al, 1993). This protein is also a major autoantigen in primary biliary cirrhosis (Fussey et al, 1988). The prosthetic group of this protein, lipoic acid, is covalently bound to the e-nitrogen of a lysine residue. Lipoic acid can inhibit the recognition of the 52 kDa protein and the trifluoroacetyl protein adducts, indicating that the 52 kDa protein, lipoic acid and trifluoro-acetylated proteins have similar three-dimensional structures, resulting in molecular mimicry.

AUTOIMMUNE HEPATITIS (AIH) TYPE 2

Autoimmune hepatitis is a rare autoimmune disease which is estimated to be found in 20–30 cases per million of the population. AIH is characterized by a marked female predominance (female:male ratio 4:1), hyper-gammaglobulinaemia, circulating autoantibodies, benefit from immuno-suppression, extrahepatic clinical autoimmune syndromes and an over-representation of patients with the immunogenetic background of HLA B8, DR3 or DR4 (Johnson and McFarlane, 1993) (Table 1). According to the autoantibodies found, patients with autoimmune hepatitis are further subdivided into AIH types 1–3 (Table 2). AIH type 2 is characterized by the presence of LKM autoantibodies. These autoantibodies were first described by Rizzetto, using the method of indirect immunofluorescence on rodent liver and kidney sections. Their characteristic feature is the exclusive staining of the P3 portion of the proximal renal tubules (Rizzetto et al, 1973). Western blots with hepatic microsomes revealed a protein band of 50 kDa. In addition to the 50 kDa protein, a 55 kDa and a 74 kDa protein are detected at a lower frequency (Codoner-Franch et al, 1989; Manns et al, 1989). Two independent approaches led to P450 2D6 as the major antigen of LKM1 autoantibodies. The first approach involved screening of human liver cDNA libraries and the identification of P450 2D6 by sequence analysis (Guenguen et al, 1989; Manns et al, 1989). The second approach used the specific inhibition of the enzymatic activity of the target protein for identification, demonstrating that LKM1 autoantibodies inhibit the hydroxylation of bufuralol, a substrate of P450 2D6 in isolated liver microsomes (Zanger et al, 1988). This inhibition was confirmed later in vitro with sparteine metabolism, an antiarrhythmic drug (Manns et al, 1990a). In contrast to bufuralol, sparteine can be used in vivo as a test substrate for P450 2D6-mediated metabolism (Manns et al 1990a). At the time of liver biopsy sparteine was used in order to characterize the in vivo phenotype of the patients. Cytochrome P450 2D6 in humans is subject to a pronounced polymorphism. Some 5–10% of the population are devoid a functional cytochrome P450 2D6, resulting in a low metabolizer phenotype for the major substrates of the enzyme, for example, debrisoquine (Gonzalez et al, 1988). Therefore this test series, which was later confirmed with a second series that included more than 50 patients (Manns, unpublished), revealed two results. First, all patients with LKM-positive autoimmune hepatitis type 2 included in this series were extensive metabolizers of sparteine, expressing functional P450 2D6 protein. Therefore the low-metabolizer phenotype does not predispose to AIH type 2. Second, LKM1 auto-antibodies do inhibit P450 2D6 activity in vitro but not in vivo (Manns et al 1990a). Finally, the expression of P450 2D6 seems to be a prerequisite for the development of LKM1 autoantibodies directed against P450 2D6.

The structures recognized by LKM autoantibodies were further characterized. Manns et al tested a total of 26 LKM-positive sera using Western blotting of partial sequences of recombinant cytochrome P450 2D6. Of these sera, 11 recognized a short minimal epitope of eight amino acids. The amino acid sequence of this minimal epitope is DPAQPPRD (Figure 10). Twelve other clones recognized a sequence comprising 15–33 amino acids, and four clones recognized the C-terminal two-thirds of P450 2D6. Searching the EMBL data base with the minimal epitope revealed a striking match with the primary structure of the immediate early protein IE 175 of HSV-1. Sequence identity is seen for the sequence PAQPPR. Therefore the LKM1 autoantibodies were affinity-purified against P450 2D6 and used in Western blots with lysates of BHK cells infected with HSV. Interestingly the autoantibody specifically detected a band at 175 kDa, demonstrating cross-reactivity of at least some LKM1 sera with an HSV-specific protein of 175 kDa. The hypothesis that molecular mimicry might contribute to autoantibody formation at least in some cases of AIH was suggested on the basis of a case study. In a pair of identical twins, one sister suffers from AIH type 2, and the other one is healthy. Interestingly, only the sister suffering from AIH is HSV-positive, and her serum recognizes the

Linear epitopes on P450 2D6 in autoimmune hepatitis type 2

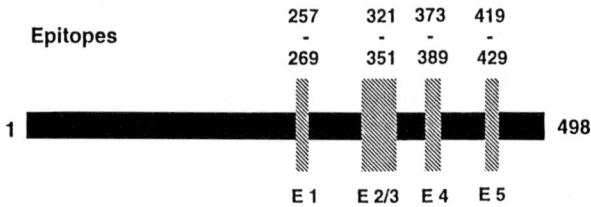

Epitope	Sequence	% Recognition
E1	257 - 269	90
E2/3	321 - 351	80
E4	373 - 389	8
E5	419 - 429	8

Figure 10. Linear B-cell epitopes on P450 2D6 in autoimmune hepatitis type 2. Modified from Yamamoto et al (1993b).

viral 175 kDa protein in lysates of HSV-infected cells. Molecular mimicry might contribute to the development of AIH by weakening self-tolerance to certain protein targets; however, for AIH, HSV infection cannot account for most of the cases of AIH studied. First, not all patients with AIH were HSV-positive, and second, most LKM1-positive sera need a larger epitope for reaction. The additional sequence, however, is derived from P450 2D6 and is quite different from IE 175 (Manns et al, 1991).

Further work on epitope mapping was performed by Yamamoto, resulting in the identification of three other epitopes on P450 2D6. They confirmed that most patients with AIH recognize the epitope of amino acids 257–269, including the core sequence of DPAQPPRD. However, about 50% of AIH patients in addition recognized an epitope from amino acids 321–351 and some cases recognized an epitope of amino acids 373–389 or 410–429 (Figure 10) (Yamamoto et al, 1993b).

Next to these linear epitopes, recent work suggests the presence of conformational autoantibodies. Absorption studies of LKM1 sera were performed using peptides of the four domains described by Yamamoto to pre-absorb the sera. The pre-absorbed sera were used for inhibition of P450 2D6-mediated enzyme reactions. While most of the inhibitory activity of the autoantibodies could not be abolished by saturating binding-sites for the linear peptides, affinity-purified autoantibodies directed against these linear epitopes also failed significantly to inhibit the P450 2D6-mediated enzymatic activity. The authors conclude that the inhibitory activity is due to the presence of conformational autoantibodies (Duclos-Vallee et al, 1995). As multiple epitopes are recognized by most of the patient's sera, it was proposed that the original immune response may be polyclonal and that it develops later into an oligoclonal response by affinity maturation. The immunodominant sites are believed to be due to the structural and sequential characteristics of the protein and the genetic background of the patient (Yamamoto et al, 1993b).

In about 10% of patients with autoimmune hepatitis a protein band of 55 kDa, the LKM3 autoantibody, is detected. Due to the low abundance of this autoantibody, we were able to test only five sera with LKM3 auto-antibodies. In four patients sera LKM3 was associated with LKM1 autoantibodies; one patient, however, was positive only for LKM3. Epitope mapping revealed a minimal epitope from amino acids 264–373, indicating that the autoantibody is conformation-dependent (Straub et al, 1994).

Today, LKM1 autoantibodies are widely used as diagnostic markers for AIH or autoimmunity associated with hepatitis C. However, the patho-genetic role of these autoantibodies is not known. One possible mech-anism of liver injury mediated by these autoantibodies could be that mediated by direct binding of LKM autoantibodies to the hepatocytes. Such a binding event would result in lysis of hepatocytes either by complement or by antibody-directed cell-mediated cytotoxicity (ADCC). A prerequisite for the activation of both mechanisms is the surface expres-sion of P450 2D6. As discussed earlier for tienilic acid-induced hepatitis, there are controversial results concerning the presence of cytochromes P450 in the plasma membrane. However, two very carefully controlled investigations demonstrate that cytochromes P450 are located on the surface of the ER membrane, indicating that LKM autoantibodies might participate in the pathogenesis of autoimmune hepatitis (Loeper et al, 1993; Robin et al, 1995)

Cellular immune response to cytochrome P450 2D6

Tissue-infiltrating T-lymphocytes are major components of piecemeal necrosis. This finding implies that T-lymphocytes might play a major role in the pathogenic processes leading to cell damage and inflammation. In order to investigate whether T-cells react to the same antigens recognized by LKM autoantibodies, Löhr and coworkers prepared 189 T-cell clones isolated from liver biopsies of four different patients with autoimmune hepatitis type 2. These clones were isolated with limiting dilution and propagated in vitro by recombinant IL-2. Four of these clones proliferated specifically in response to human recombinant cytochrome P450 2D6. These T lymphocytes were of the T-helper phenotype and were inhibited by MHC class II monoclonal antibodies (Löhr et al, 1991).

Regulation of cytochromes P450 during liver regeneration

In order to investigate the regulation of the target of autoimmunity under conditions of regeneration and in the presence of acute phase markers, Trautwein performed a series of experiments (Trautwein et al, 1992; Trautwein et al, personal communication). First he investigated how cytochrome P450 2D6 is regulated under the influence of acute-phase mediators: IL-1, IL-6 and TNFα. All of these acute-phase mediators reduced the levels of cytochrome P450 2D6 expression: IL-1 and TNF-α resulted in a 4-fold reduction 6 hours after intraperitoneal injection, while only a mild reduction of P450 2D6 was seen after application of IL-6. Further investigations were done to see how cytochromes P450 are regulated during liver regeneration. Two-thirds hepatectomy was performed, and levels of RNA, protein and enzymatic activity were measured for cytochromes P450 1A2, 2E1 and 3A. These results revealed a transient down-regulation of cytochromes P450 1A2 and P450 2E1 after liver hepatectomy on the RNA level. The expression of P450 3A, however, remained unaffected. Due to the long half-lives of cytochromes P450 the down-regulation on the RNA level was too short to be translated into a significant reduction of P450 protein. In spite of constant protein levels, the enzymatic activity of P450 2E1 decreased significantly, indicating that during liver regeneration cytochrome P450 activity is also regulated on the post-translational level. These results indicate that, during prolonged phases with ongoing liver regeneration and the presence of acute-phase mediators, cytochromes P450 are likely to be down-regulated on the RNA, protein and the activity levels. Therefore, a higher susceptibility of patients to drug-induced toxicity might be expected, and medication should be applied with great care.

Genetics of AIH

It is well accepted that AIH type 1 is associated with the HLA-A1-B8-DR3 haplotype in the white population (Mackay and Morris, 1972; Freudenberg et al, 1977; Tait et al, 1989; Donaldson et al, 1991; Scully et al, 1993). The relative risk of people bearing this haplotype was reported to be 12 (Wittingham et al, 1981). The closest association exists with DR3. Linkage equilibrium between the HLA-DR3 and the HLA-B8 loci exists and contributes to the association of AIH type 1 with the B8 haplotype (Mackay and Morris, 1972; Tait et al, 1989; Mackay, 1991). In England, in the DR3-negative population, a significant increase of DR4 is noted, suggesting that DR4 is a second independent risk factor in white people (Donaldson et al, 1991). Patients with the HLA-A1-B8 haplotype have a lower age of onset of the disease, relapse after treatment more frequently, and need transplantation more often compared to patients with the DR-4 haplotype (Donaldson et al, 1991).

The situation is different in Japan, where AIH type 1 is rare. In Japanese patients no association with HLA-DR3 is found. However, an association with HLA-DR4 is observed with a relative risk of developing AIH type 1 of 14.8 (Seki et al, 1990). Further, a highly significant association of AIH type 1 was found for HLA-B54, with a frequency of this allele of 45.2% in patients with AIH as compared to 10.9% in controls (Seki et al, 1990). However, neither in the white nor in the Japanese population were serological markers associated with the genetic background identified. Further, AIH type 1 is associated with C4A gene deletions responsible for an increase of the C4A-Q0 alleles (Vergani et al, 1985; Scully et al, 1993). The significance of this finding is unknown; however, C4 is known to be involved in immune complex clearance and might indicate that a viral agent might be involved in the pathogenesis of the disease.

In LKM1 antibody-positive autoimmune hepatitis, preliminary results of our group and others also indicate an association with HLA DR-3 and C4A-Q0 (Lenzi et al, 1992; Manns and Krüger, 1994).

AUTOIMMUNE HEPATITIS AS PART OF THE AUTO-IMMUNE POLYGLANDULAR SYNDROME TYPE 1 (APS1)

Autoimmune polyendocrine syndrome type 1 (APS1) is a rare autosomal recessive disorder, characterized by a variable combination of disease components (Neufeld et al, 1980; Ahonen et al, 1990; Riley, 1992). The first clinical manifestation of APS1 usually occurs in childhood, and progressively new components may appear throughout life, the majority (63%) of the patients suffering from three to five of them (Ahonen et al, 1990). The most frequent components in APS1 are chronic mucocutaneous candidiasis, hypoparathyroidism, adrenocortical failure and gonadal failure in females (Neufeld et al, 1980; Ahonen et al, 1990; Riley, 1992). Auto-immune hepatitis is a serious but less frequent disease component (Neufeld et al, 1980; Ahonen et al, 1990; Riley, 1992). In contrast to other auto-immune diseases, female predominance and linkage to the HLA-DR haplo-type do not exist (Ahonen et al, 1990). The APS1 locus has been assigned to the long arm of chromosome 21 (Aaltonen et al, 1994). Lymphocytic infiltration of the affected organs and the presence of organ-specific auto-antibodies are typical features of APS1 (Arulantham et al, 1979).

Recently, progress was made in the study of APS1-related Addison's disease, which affects more than 60% of APS1 patients (Neufeld et al, 1980; Ahonen et al, 1990; Riley, 1992). Adrenal autoantigens in APS1 are cytochromes P450 c17, P450 scc and P450 c21, which are all enzymes involved in steroidogenesis (Krohn et al, 1992; Winqvist et al, 1992, 1994, 1995; Peterson and Krohn, 1994; Uibo et al, 1994a, b; Song et al, 1994). P450 c21 is reported to be present in the adrenal cortex, expression of P450 c17 is found in adrenal tissue and steroid-producing cells of testis and ovary, and P450 scc is expressed in adrenals, in gonads and in placenta (Uibo et al, 1994a). Autoantibodies directed against adrenal and ovarian tissue are of high predictive value: they are often present for several years preceeding failure of these organs (Ahonen et al, 1987).

Chronic hepatitis is a serious disease component present in 10–18% of patients with APS1 (Neufeld et al, 1980; Ahonen et al, 1990; Riley, 1992), and occasional deaths related to hepatitis are reported to occur in APS1 without signs of pre-warning (Ahonen et al, 1990; Michele et al 1994). Recently we succeeded in identifying the first hepatic autoantigen in autoimmune hepatitis related to APS1 (Clemente et al 1995). The patient serum was characterized by a predominant staining of the peri-venous hepatocytes. This pattern differs from the homogeneous staining pattern found in patients with isolated autoimmune hepatitis, suggesting that the patient serum recognizes an autoantigen that is different from LKM1 (anti-cytochrome P450 2D6) and LKM3 (anti-UDP-glucuronosyltransferase) autoantibodies, which, as described earlier, are targets for autoimmunity in patients with autoimmune and virus hepatitis (Manns et al, 1990b; Philipp et al, 1994). Western blots with recombinant cytochromes P450s revealed that cytochrome P450 1A2 is the target of this autoantigen. This result retrospectively identified 'an unusual case of autoimmune hepatitis' (Sacher et al, 1990; Manns et al, 1990a) which was reported before by our group. This patient suffered from vitiligo, alopecia, nail dystrophy and had a brother who died from Addison's disease. In accordance with the criteria for diagnosis of APS1 from Neufeld this patient suffered from APS1 (Neufeld et al, 1980). These two cases of AIH clearly demonstrate that in APS-1 related hepatitis at least one important target autoantigen is cytochrome P450 1A2, which was known before to be the target antigen in dihydralazine hepatitis, where it is subject to adduct formation with an activated metabolite of the drug. This adduct formation probably results in the immunization against this self-antigen (Beaune et al, 1994). In contrast in patients with APS1 no relationship between P450 1A2 and drug usage is known. The underlying immune defect and the pathogenetic mechanisms remain to be determined. However, due to the relatively high frequency of hepatitis in patients with APS1, constant monitoring of autoantibody status and specific reactivity of T-cells might provide further insights in the course of the disease and the underlying mechanisms.

VIRUS ASSOCIATED AUTOIMMUNITY

Chronic hepatitis C

Chronic infection with hepatitis C is known to induce autoimmune reactions. Hepatitis C is associated with an array of extrahepatic mani-festations, including mixed cryoglobulinaemia; membrano-proliferative glomerulonephritis, polyarthritis, porphyria cutanea tarda, Sjörgen's syndrome and autoimmune thyroid disease (Ferri et al, 1991; Agnello et al, 1992; Cacoub et al, 1992; Fargion et al, 1992; Haddad et al, 1992; DeCastro et al, 1993; Johnson et al, 1993; Tran et al, 1993). Not surprisingly, numerous autoantibodies are found to be associated with chronic hepatitis C (e.g. ANA, SMA, LKM or anti-thyroid antibodies (Bianchi et al, 1993). An HCV-specific autoantibody was found with anti-GOR that is present in at least 80% of sera from patients with HCV hepatitis. The epitope recognized by anti-GOR is GRRGQKAKSNPNRPL. It is located on a nuclear protein that is overexpressed in hepatocellular carcinoma (Mishiro et al, 1990). Interestingly, anti-GOR is not associated with autoimmune hepatitis, but is specific for hepatitis induced by HCV (Michel et al, 1992).

Depending on the geographical origin, a variable proportion of patients with LKM1 antibody-associated liver disease are-infected with HCV. The prevalence of HCV infection among LKM1-positive patients is about 90% in Japan and Italy (Lenzi et al, 1991; Miyachi, personal communication), about 50% in France and Germany (Lunel et al, 1992; Michel et al, 1992) and less than 10% in England (Lenzi et al; 1991). LKM1-positive patient populations with and without HCV are clinically different, implicating a pathogenic role for HCV in the pathogenesis of the disease (Lunel et al, 1992; Michel et al, 1992). HCV-negative patients show a pathogenesis typical for autoimmune hepatitis. They have a low age of onset, 80% of patients are female, they have a high inflammatory activity and show a good response to immunosuppression (Table 4). In contrast, the LKM-positive patients with hepatitis C have a very different pathogenesis. The age of onset is above 40 years, inflammatory activity is low, response to corticosteroids is not convincing and the majority of these patients do not require treatment because disease activity is low (Table 4).

Further characterization of LKM autoantibodies revealed differences between LKM1 autoantibodies in AIH and in hepatitis C. Most of the LKM-positive sera from patients with AIH are positive in Western blot and recognize small linear epitopes of P450 2D6. However, in HCV-positive patients a more heterogeneous autoimmune reaction is found. Several research groups demonstrated that, in hepatitis C, only about 30% of the sera reveal a band of 50 kDa in Western blots (Ma et al 1992; Yamamoto et al, 1993c; Durazzo et al, 1995). Additional bands were detected at 59 kDa and 70 kDa; however, not more than 45% of patients' sera were found to react at all in Western blots (Durazzo et al, 1995). In spite of the low frequency of detection of the LKM1 antigen in Western blots, a significant proportion of Western blot-negative sera were found to be LKM1-positive by a specific LKM1 ELISA. These sera contain conformation-dependent LKM1 autoantibodies, since denaturation of the antigens prior to ELISA testing resulted in a total loss of the signal (Durazzo et al, 1995). A possible association of the induction of LKM autoantibodies and a specific HCV strain was investigated. HCV genotype 2 was found to be the predominant strain in Italian and German patients with chronic hepatitis C and auto-immunity to LKM antigens. Because some sequence homology between HCV and P450 2D6 exists in the core, the envelope and the NS5 regions of HCV the regions with high homology were amplified and sequenced; however, no sequence changes increasing the homology between P450 2D6

Table 4. Comparison of AIH type 2 and hepatitis C associated with LKM autoantibodies.

	Autoimmune hepatitis type 2 with LKM1 autoantibodies	Chronic hepatitis C associated with LKM1 autoantibodies
Age of onset	Young	Older
Sex	80% female	No prevalence
ALT	+++	+
LKM titre	+++	+
Benefit from immunosuppression	+++	None
Benefit from interferon treatment	Harmful	(+)
HLA-DR3	+++	+
C4A-Q0	+++	+++
Anti-HCV antibodies, HCV-RNA	–	+

and HCV could be detected. The production of LKM autoantibodies is also not related to a specific genotype of HCV (Michitaka et al, 1994).

Chronic hepatitis D

In their original report, Crivelli et al (1983) observed that 11/81 patients with chronic hepatitis D had serum antibodies directed against hepatic microsomes and the proximal renal tubules. The reaction was strongest if human and primate tissues were used, and progressively declined from ox to pig to rabbit and to rat. In contrast to LKM1 and LKM2 autoantibodies, which react with liver and kidney tissues only, additional fluorescence was detected with pancreas, adrenal gland, thyroid and stomach. The newly defined autoantibody was called LKM3. It is further distinguished from LKM1 and LKM2 autoantibodies by the molecular weight of the target antigen, which is about 55 kDa. The molecular target of the LKM3 auto-antibody was identified by screening a cDNA library. Screening of a cDNA library and subsequent sequence analysis of the positive clone revealed UGT 1.6 as a target of the LKM 3 autoantibody (Philipp et al, 1994). Therefore Western blotting with recombinant rabbit UGT 1.6 was used to characterize the clinical significance of LKM3 autoantibodies. LKM3 auto-antibodies were detected only in patients with hepatitis D and patients with autoimmune hepatitis. They were not detected in sera from patients with hepatitis B, hepatitis C, primary biliary cirrhosis, primary sclerosing cholangitis or lupus erythematosus.

UGTs are encoded in a large gene cluster (Figure 3). At least six different exons 1 are connected to the constant exons 2–5 by differential splicing. Testing LKM3 autoantibodies with several family 1 UGTs revealed reactivity to UGT 1.1, UGT 1.4 and UGT 1.6 in all sera tested. As exons 1 differ between all these UGTs, this result indicates that the epitope is located in the C-terminal part of family 1 UGTs. Epitope mapping experiments confirmed that most sera recognized the C-terminus alone. However, the signal obtained with the sera was very weak and disappeared if the C-terminus was further truncated. The signal was much higher if some N-terminal sequence was included in the clones, resulting in a minimal epitope of amino acids 264–373. As truncation from the C-terminus, the N-terminus or central deletions resulted in a total loss of reactivity, it can be concluded that the epitope is conformation-dependent (Straub et al, 1994). In addition to the major epitope on family 1 UGTs, a minor epitope was found on UGT 2B13. This epitope was recognized by 2/8 LKM3-positive patient sera with HDV and the signal was much lower than signals detected with UGT family 1 (Philipp et al, 1994). With the detection of UGTs for the first time, a drug-metabolizing enzyme of phase 2 was identified as an autoantigen.

In contrast to cytochromes P450, which are expressed on the cytoplasmic site of the ER, UGTs are luminal ER proteins. These proteins should be expected to be located on the outer membrane of the ER, if transported to the surface via Golgi. Further work is needed to investigate the surface expression of UGT1 in hepatocytes and to correlate the presence of LKM3 autoantibodies and the titres of LKM3 in the serum with the pathogenesis of HDV infection.

DISCUSSION

Significant progress has been made in recent years concerning the molecular identification of hepatocellular autoantigens. For autoimmune diseases associated with the formation of anti-liver/kidney microsomal autoantibodies, drug-metabolizing enymes were repeatedly detected as targets for autoimmunity. With the exception of drug-induced hepatitis, little is known about the aetiology of these autoimmune diseases. It remains to be determined whether autoantibodies specifically associated with these diseases can give us clues towards an aetiology, for example, via molecular mimicry between the sequence of B-cell epitopes of these auto-antigenes and infectious agents. Furthermore, it needs to be determined whether the T-cell response is directed against the same target proteins. The characterization of the T-cell response will also provide insight in the mechanisms involved in the aetiology of these diseases and will reveal potential defects and abnormalities in the regulation of immune response and the cytokine pattern in these patients.

Currently autoantibodies are used as diagnostic tools which help us to identify subsets of patients who share a common response towards specific treatment, for example, immunosuppressive agents, interferons or bile acids. Furthermore, particular autoantibodies, such as LKM1 and LKM3, occur in association with a subset of patients with hepatitis C or D. It remains to be investigated whether these autoantibodies contribute to tissue damage and, hence, cause the disease to follow a more severe course. Further, LKM auto-antibodies in viral hepatitis may identify patients with a particular response to treatment, for example, interferon versus corticosteroids.

Patients with APS1 who suffer from a multitude of autoimmune manifestations may present a model system for the development of autoimmune diseases. As these patients develop new manifestations of autoimmunity throughout their lifetime, B- and T-cell responses against known molecular targets of autoimmunity should be continuously monitored. First, the patients may profit directly from the study, being closely monitored and treated early in the developement of new disease components; second, changes in B- and T-cell activity would be monitored as the novel disease component develops. Knowing the immunological aberrations involved in APS1 may help to develop concepts for the treatment of this autoimmune disease and to develop concepts for the aetiology of organ-specific auto-immune diseases, for example, autoimmune hepatitis.

SUMMARY

Autoantibodies directed against cytochromes P450 or UDP-glucuronosyl-transferases (UGTs) are detected in hepatitis of different aetiology:

drug-induced hepatitis autoimmune hepatitis type 2, hepatitis associated with the autoimmune polyglandular syndrome type 1 (APS1) and virus-induced autoimmunity. Autoantibodies directed against cytochrome P450 2C9 are induced by tienilic acid, and anti-P450 1A2 autoantibodies by dihydralazine. Potential mechanisms involved may be metabolic activation of the drugs by cytochromes P450, adduct formation and circumvention of T cell tolerance. In contrast, little is known about the aetiology of auto-immune hepatitis type 2. This disease is characterized by marked female predominance, hypergammaglobulinaemia, circulating autoantibodies and benefit from immunosuppression. Patients with HLA B8, DR3 or DR4 are over-represented. The major target of autoimmunity in this disease is cytochrome P450 2D6. The autoantibodies were shown to be directed against at four short linear epitopes. In addition, about 10% of the patient sera form an additional autoantibody that detects a conformational epitope on UGTs of family 1. The phenomenon of virus-associated autoimmunity is found in chronic infections with hepatitis C and D. In chronic hepatitis C the major target of the autoantibodies again is cytochrome P450 2D6. Some linear and a high proportion of conformational epitopes are recognized. The LKM3 autoantibody is found in 13% of patients with chronic hepatitis D. The target proteins are UGTs of family 1 and, in some sera also, low titres of anto-antibodies directed against UGTs of family 2 are found. The epitopes detected are conformational. In contrast to the patients suffering from autoimmune hepatitis, patients with hepatitis as part of the auto-immune polyglandular syndrome type 1 recognize cytochrome P450 1A2. Interestingly, in APS1 patients also, autoantibodies directed against cytochromes P450 c21, P450 scc and P450 c17a may be detected; these autoantibodies are associated with adrenal and ovarian failure.

Acknowledgement

This work was supported by the Deutsch Forschungsgemeinschaft grant SFB 244.

REFERENCES

Aaltonen J, Bjorses P, Sadkuijl L et al (1994) An autosomal locus causing autoimmune disease: autoimmune polyglandular disease type 1 assigned to chromosome 21. *Nature Genetics* **8:** 83–87.

Agnello V, Chung RT & Kaplan L (1992) A role of hepatitis C virus infection in type II cryoglobulin-emia. *New England Journal of Medicine* **19:** 1490.

Ahonen P, Miettinen A & Perheentupa J (1987) Adrenal and steroidal cell antibodies in patients with autoimmune polyglandular disease type I and risk of adrenocortical and ovarian failure. *Journal of Clinical Endocrinology and Metabolism* **64:** 494–500.

Ahonen P, Koskimies S, Lokki ML et al (1988) The expression of autoimmune polyglandular disease type I appears associated with several HLA-A antigens but not with HLA-DR. *Journal of Clinical Endocrinology and Metabolism* **66:** 1152–1157.

Ahonen P, Myllärniemi S, Sipilä I & Perheentupa J (1990) Clinical variation of autoimmune poly-endocrinopathy-candidiasis-ectodermal dystrophy (APECED) in a series of 68 patients. *New England Journal of Medicine* **322:** 1829–1836.

Arulantham K, Dwyer JM, Genel M et al (1979) Evidence for defective immunoregulation in the syndrome of familial candidiasis endocrinopathy. *New England Journal of Medicine* **300:** 164–168.

Beaune PH, Bourdi M, Belloc C et al (1993) Immunotoxicology and expression of human cytochrome P450 in microorganisms. *Toxicology* **82:** 53–60.

Beaune PH, Pessayre D, Dansette P et al (1994) Autoantibodies against cytochromes P450: role in human diseases. *Advances in Pharmacology* **30:** 199–245.

Bernuau J, Mallet L & Benhamon JP (1981) Hepatotoxicite due a l'acide tienilique. *Gastroenterologie Clinique et Biologique* **5:** 692–693.

Bianchi FB, Lenzi, Cassani F et al (1993) Immunology and autoimmunity in hepatis C. In Meyer zum Büschenfelde KH, Hoofnagle J, Manns M (eds) *Immunology and the Liver*. pp 102–104. Dordrecht: Kluwer Academic Publishers.

Boccaccio F, Attali P, Nataf J et al (1987) Hepatite aigue a la dihydralazine. *Gastroenterologie Clinique et Biologique* **11:** 614.

Bock KW (1992) Metabolic polymorphisms affecting activation of toxic and mutagenic arylamines. *Trends in Pharmacological Science* **13:** 223–226.

Bourdi M, Larrey D, Nataf J et al (1990) Anti-liver endoplasmatic reticulum autoantibodies are directed against human cytochrome P450 IA2: a specific marker of dihydralazine-induced hepatitis. *Journal of Clinical Investigation* **85:** 1967–1973.

Bourdi M, Gautier JC, Micheva J et al (1992) Anti-liver microsomes autoantibodies and dihydralazune induced hepatitis: specificity of autoantibodies and inductive capacity of the drug. *Molecular Pharmacology* **42:** 280–285.

Bourdi M, Tinel M, Beaune PH & Pessayre D (1994) Interactions of dihydralazine with cytochromes P4501A: a possible explanation for the appearance of anti-P450 1A2 autoantibodies. *Molecular Pharmacology* **45:** 1287–1295.

Burchell B, Nebert DW, Nelson DR et al (1991) The UDP-glucuronosyltransferase gene superfamily: suggested nomenclature based on evolutionary divergence. *DNA and Cell Biology* **10:** 487–494.

Burchell B, Coughtree MWH & Jansen PLM (1994) Function and regulation of UDP-glucuronosyltransferase genes in health and liver disease: report on the seventh international workshop on glucuronidation, September 1993, Pitlochry, Scotland. *Hepatology* **20:** 1622–1630.

Butler LE, Thomassen D, Martin JL et al (1992) The calcium binding protein calreticulin is covalently modified in rat liver by a reactive metabolite of the inhalation anaesthetic halothane. *Chemical Research in Toxicology* **5:** 406–410.

Cacoub P, Lunel-Fabiani F, Huong Du LT et al (1992) Polyarteritis nodosa and hepatitis C infection. *Annals of Internal Medicine* **116:** 605–606.

Christen U, Jeno P & Gut J (1993) Halothane metabolism: the dihydrolipoamide acetyltransferase subunit of the pyruvate dehydrogenase complex mimics trifluoroacetyl-protein adducts. *Biochemistry* **32:** 1492–1499.

Clemente MG, Obermayer-Straub P, Meloni A et al (1995) Autoantibodies against cytochrome P450 1A2 in a patient with liver disease in autoimmune polyendocrine syndrome type 1. 30th Annual Meeting of the German Association of the Study of the Liver, Kopenhagen. *Journal of Hepatology* (in press).

Codoner-Franch P, Paradis P, Guenguen M et al (1989) A new antigen recognized by anti-liver-microsome antibody (LKMA). *Clinical and Experimental Immunology* **159:** 542–547.

Crivelli O, Lavarini C, Chiaberge E et al (1983) Microsomal autoantibodies in chronic infection with HBsAg associated delta (d) agent. *Clinical and Experimental Immunology* **54:** 232–238.

DeCastro M, Sanchez J, Herrera JF et al (1993) Hepatitis C virus antibodies and liver disease in patients with porphyria cutanea tarda. *Hepatology* **17:** 551–557.

De Lemos-Chiarandini C, Alvarez F, Bernard O et al (1987a) Determination of the membrane topology of the phenobarbital-inducible rat liver cytochrome P450 isoenzyme PB-4 using site-specific antibodies. *Journal of Cell Biology* **104:** 209–219.

De Lemos-Chiarandini C, Alvarez F et al (1987b) Anti-Liver-Kidney microsome antibody is a marker for the rat hepatocyte endoplasmic reticulum Hepatology **7:** 468–475.

Dienstag IL (1990) Hepatitis non-A, non-B: C at last. *Gastroenterology* **99:** 1177–1180.

Donaldson PT, Doherty DG, Hayliar KM et al (1991) Susceptibility to autoimmune chronic active hepatitis: human leukocyte antigens DR 4 and A1-B8-Dr-3 are independent risk factors. *Hepatology* **13:** 701–706.

Duclos-Vallee JC, Hajoui O, Yamamoto AM, Jacqz-Aigrain E & Alvarez F (1995) Conformational epitopes on Cyp 2D6 are recognized by liver/kidney microsomal antibodies. *Gastroenterology* **108:** 470–476.

Durazzo M, Philipp T, van Pelt FNAM et al (1995) Heterogeneity of microsomal autoantibodies (LKM) in chronic hepatitis C and D virus infection. *Gastroenterology* **108:** 455–462.

Fargion S, Peperno A, Cappellini MD et al (1992) Hepatitis C virus and porphyria cutanea tarda: evidence of a strong association. *Hepatology* **16:** 1322–1326.

Eade OE, Grice D, Krawit EL et al (1981) HLA A and b locus antigens in patients with unexplained hepatitis following halothane anaesthesia. *Tissue Antigens* **17:** 428–432.

Ferri C, Greco F, Longombardo G et al (1991) association between hepatitis C virus and mixed cryo-globulinemia. *Clinical and Experimental Rheumatology* **9:** 621–624.

Fevery J (1981) Pathogenesis of Gilbert's syndrome. *European Journal of Clinical Investigations* **11:** 417–418.

Freudenberg J, Baumann H, Arnold W et al (1977) HLA in different forms of chronic active hepatitis: a comparison between adult patients and children. *Digestion* **15:** 260–270.

Fussey SPM, Guest JR, James OFW et al (1988) Identification and analysis of the major autoantigens in primary biliary cirrhosis. *Proceedings of the National Academy of Science of the USA* **85:** 8654–8658.

Gonzalez FJ, Skoda RC, Kimura S et al (1988) Characterization of the common genetic defect in humans deficient in debrisoquine metabolism. *Nature* **331:** 442–446.

Gruenke LD, Konopka DR & Koop Drand Waskell LA (1988) Characterization of halothane oxidation by hepatic microsomes and purified cytochrome P450 using gas chromatographic mass spectometric assay. *Journal of Pharmacological and Experimental Therapies* **246:** 454–459.

Guengerich FP (1993) Cytochrome P450 enzymes. *American Scientist* **81:** 440–447.

Guenguen M, Yamamoto AM, Bernd O & Alvarez F (1989) Anti-liver kidney microsome antibody type 1 recognizes human cytochrome P450 db1. *Biochemical and Biophysical Research Communications* **159:** 542–547.

Gut J, Christen U, Huwyler J et al (1992) Molecular mimicry of trifluoroacetylated human liver protein adducts by constitutive proteins and immunochemical evidence for its impairment in halothane hepatitis. *European Journal of Biochemistry* **210:** 569–576.

Gut J, Christen U & Huwyler J (1993) Mechanisms of halothane toxicity: novel insights. *Pharmacological Therapy* **58:** 133–158.

Haddad J, Deny P, Munz-Gotheil C et al (1992) Lymphocyticsialadenitis of Sjörgen's syndrome associated with chronic hepatitis c virus liver disease. *Lancet* **339:** 321–323.

Hoft RH, Bunker JP, Goodman HI & Gregory PB (1981) Halothane hepatitis in three pairs of closely related women. *New England Journal of Medicine* **304:** 1023–1024.

Homberg JC, Andre C & Abuaf N (1984) A new anit-liver/kidney-microsome antibody (anti-LKM2) in tienilic induced hepatitis. *Clinical and Experimental Immunology* **55:** 561–570.

Homberg JC, Abuaf N, Hemly-Khalid et al (1985) Drug induced hepatitis associated with anticyto-plasmic organelle autoantibodies. *Hepatology* **5:** 722–725.

Iyanagi T, Haniu M, Sogawa K et al (1986) Cloning and characterization of cDNA ending methyl-cholanthrene inducible rat mRNA for UDP-glucuronosyltransferase. *Journal of Biological Chemistry* **261:** 15 607–15 614.

Jarasch ED, Kartenberg J, Bruder G et al (1979) B-types cytochromes in plasma membrane isolated from rat liver, in comparison with those from endomembranes. *Journal of Cell Biology* **80:** 37–52.

Johnson RJ & McFarlane IG (1993) Meeting report: international autoimmune hepatitis group. *Hepatology* **18:** 998–1005.

Johnson RJ, Gretch DR, Yamabe et al (1993) Membranoproliferative glomerulonephritis associated with hepatitis C virus infection. *New England Journal of Medicine* **18:** 465–470.

Kenna JG & van Pelt FNAM (1994) The metabolism and toxicity of inhaled anaesthetic agents. *Anaesthetical and Pharmacological Reviews* **2:** 29–42.

Kenna JG, Martin JL, Satoh H & Pohl LR (1990a) Purification of trifluoroacetylated protein antigens from livers of halothane-treated rats. *European Journal of Pharmacology* **183:** 1139–1140.

Kenna JG, Martin JL, Satoh H & Pohl LR (1990b) Factors affecting the expression of trifluoro-acetylated liver microsomal protein neoantigens in rats treated with halothane. *Drug Metabolism and Disposition* **18:** 788–793.

Knights KM, Gourlay GK, Gibson RA & Cousins MJ (1988) Halothane induced hepatic necrosis in rats. The role of in vivo lipid peroxiodation. *Pharmacology and Toxicology* **63:** 327–332.

Koop DR (1992) Oxidative and reductive metabolism by cytochrome P450 2E1. *FASEB Journal* **6:** 724–730.

Krohn K, Uibo R, Aavik E et al (1992) Identification by molecular cloning of an autoantigen associated with Addison's Disease as steroid 17a-hydroxylase. *Lancet* **339:** 770–773.

Kunze, KD, Porst H & Tschöppel L (1985) Morphologie und Pathogenese von Leberschäden durch Dihydralazin, Propanolol und Ketophenylbutazon. *Zentralblatt der Allgemeinen Pathologie und Anatomie* **130:** 509–518.

Lecoeur S, Bonierbale E, Challine D et al (1994) Specificity of in vitro covalent binding of tienilic acid metabolites to comparison with two directly hepatotoxic drugs. *Chemical Research in Toxicology* **7:** 434–442.

Lenzi M, Bianchi B, Casani F et al (1984) Liver cell surface expression of the antigen reacting with liver–kidney microsomal antibody (LKM) *Clinical and Experimental Immunology* **55:** 36–40.

Lenzi M, Johnson PJ, McFarlane IG et al (1991) Antibodies to hepatitis C virus in autoimmune liver disease; evidence for geographical heterogeneity. *Lancet* **338:** 277–280.

Lenzi M, Mantovani W, Cataleta M et al (1992) HLA typing in autoimmune hepatitis (AI-CAH) type 2. *Journal of Hepatology* **16:** 59.

Loeper J, Descartoire V, Maurice M et al (1990) Presence of functional cytochrome P450 on isolated rat hepatocyte plasma membrane. *Hepatology* **11:** 850–858.

Loeper J, Descartoire V, Maurice M et al (1993) Cytochromes P450 in human hepatocyte plasma membrane: recognition by several autoantibodies. *Gastroenterology* **104:** 203–216.

Löhr H, Manns M, Hyriasoulis et al (1991) Clonal analysis of liver infdiltrating cells in patients with chronic active hepatitis (AI-CAH). *Clinical and Experimental Immunology* **84:** 297–302.

Lopez-Garcia MP, Dansette PM, Valadon P et al (1993) Human liver P450s expressed in yeast as tools for reactive metabolite formation studies. Oxidative activation of tienilic acid by cytochrome P450 2C9 and P450 2C10. *European Journal of Biochemistry* **213:** 223–232.

Lunel F, Abuaf N, Frangeul L et al (1992) Liver-kidney microsomes antibody type 1 and hepatitis C virus infection. *Hepatology* **16:** 630–636.

Ma Y, Lenzi M, Gäken J et al (1992) The target antigen of liver kidney microsomal antibody is different in type II autoimmune chronic active hepatitis and chronic hepatitic C virus infection. *Journal of Hepatology* **16:** 4.

Mackay IR (1991) Autoimmune hepatitis: the realities and the uncertainties. *Gastroenterolerology of Japan* **28:** 102–108.

Mackay IR & Morris PJ (1972) Association of autoimmune chronic hepatitis with HLA-A1-B8. *Lancet* **ii:** 793–795.

Mackay IR & Tait BD (1980) HLA association with autoimmune type chronic active hepatitis: identification of B8-DRw3 haplotype by family studies. *Gastroenterology* **79:** 95–98.

Manns MP (1991) Cytoplasmic autoantigens in autoimmune hepatitis: molecular analysis and clinical relevance. *Seminars in Liver Disease* **11:** 205–214.

Manns M & Krüger M (1994) Genetics in liver diseases. *Gastroenterology* **106:** 1676–1697.

Manns M, Johnson EF, Griffin KJ et al (1989) The major target antigen of liver kidney microsomal autoantibodies in idiopathic autoimmune hepatitis is cytochrome P450 db1. *Journal of Clinical Investigation* **83:** 1066–1072.

Manns MP, Griffin KJ, Quattrochi L et al (1990a) Identification of cytochrome P450 IA2 as a human autoantigen. *Archives of Biochemistry and Biophysics* **280:** 229–232.

Manns M, Zanger U, Gerken G et al (1990b) Patients with type II autoimmune hepatitis express functionally intact cytochrome P450 db1 that is inhibited by LKM1 autoantibodies in vitro but not in vivo. *Hepatology* **12:** 127–132.

Manns MP, Griffin KJ, Sullivan KF & Johnson EF (1991) LKM1 autoantibodies rexcognize a short linear sequence in P450 IID6, a cytochrome P450 monooxygenase. *Journal of Clinical Investigation* **88:** 1370–1378.

Michel G, Ritter A, Gerken G et al (1992) Anti-GOR and hepatitis C virus in autoimmune liver diseases. *Lancet* **339:** 267–269.

Michele TM, Fleckenstein J, Sgrignoli AR & Tuluvath PJ (1994) Chronic active hepatitis in the type I polyglandular autoimmune syndrome. *Postgraduate Medical Journal* **70:** 128–131.

Michitaka K, Durazzo M, Tillmann H et al (1994) Analysis of hepatitis C virus genome in patients with autoimmune hepatitis type 2. *Gastroenterology* **106:** 1603–1610.

Mishiro S, Hoshi Y, Takeda K et al (1990) Non-A, non-B hepatitis specific antibodies directed at host-derived epitope: implication for an autoimmune process. *Lancet* **336:** 1400–1403.

Nataf J, Bernuau J, Larrey D et al (1986) A new anti-liver microsome antibody: a specific marker of dihydralazine-induced hepatitis. *Gastroenterology* **90:** 1751.

Nebert DW & McKinnon RA (1994) Cytochrome P450: evolution and functional diversity. *Progress in Liver Diseases* **12:** 63–97.

Nelson DR & Strobel HW (1987) The evolution of cytochrome P450 proteins. *Molecular Biology and Evolution* **4:** 572–593.

Nelson DR, Kamataki T, Waxman DJ et al (1993) The P450 superfamily: update on new sequences, gene mapping, accession numbers, early trivial names of enzymes and nomencalture. *DNA and Cell Biology* **12:** 1–51.

Neufeld M, Maclaren N & Blizzard R (1980) Autoimmune polyglandular syndromes. *Pediatric Annals* **9:** 154–162.

Paronetto F & Popper H (1970) Lymphocyte stimulation induced by halothane in patients with hepatitis following exposure to halothane. *New England Journal of Medicine* **283:** 277–280.

Pessayre D (1993) Toxic and immune mechanisms leading to acute and subacute drug induced liver injury. In Miguet JP & Dhumeaux D (eds), *Progress in Hepatology* pp 23–39. Paris: John Libbey Eurotext.

Peterson P & Krohn JE (1994) Mapping of B cell epitopes on steroid 17a-hydroxylase, an autoantigen in autoimmune polyglandular syndrome type I. *Clinical and Experimental Immunology* **98:** 104–109.

Philipp T, Durazzo M, Trautwein C et al (1994) LKM-3 autoantibodies in chronic hepatitis D recognize the UDP-glucuronosyltransferases. *Lancet* **344:** 578–581.

Plummer JL, Beckwith AJL, Bastin FN et al (1982) Free radical formation in vivo and hepatoxicity due to anaesthesia with halothane. *Anaesthesiology* **57:** 160–166.

Pohl LR, Thomassen D, Pumford NR et al (1991) Hapten carrier conjungates associated with halothane hepatitis. *Advances in Experimental and Biological Medicine* **283:** 111–120.

Pumford NR, Martin BM, Thomassen D et al (1993) Serum antibodies from halothane hepatitis patients react with the rat endoplamic reticulum protein ERp72. *Chemical Research in Toxicology* **6:** 609–615.

Ray DC & Drummond GB (1991) Halothane hepatitis. *British Journal of Anaesthesiology* **67:** 84–89.

Reinhardt M, Machnik G, Krombholz B & Jashn G (1985) Die sogenannte Dihydralazin-Hepatitis. Ein Beitrag zur Pathogenese. *Deutsche Zeitschrift der Verdauugs- und Stoffwechselkrankheiten* **45:** 283–294.

Riley WJ (1992) Autoimmune polyglandular syndromes. *Hormone Research* **38 (supplement 2):** 9–15.

Ritter JK, Chen F, Sheen YY et al (1992) A novel complex locus UGT1 encodes human bilirubin, phenol and other UDP-glucuronosyltransferase isozymes with identical carbonyl termini. *Journal of Biological Chemistry* **267:** 3257–3261.

Rizzetto M, Swana S & Doniach D (1973) Microsomal antibodies active chronic hepatitis and other disorders. *Clinical and Experimental Immunology* **15:** 331–344.

Robin MA, Maratrat M, Loeper-J et al (1995) Cytochrome P4502B follows a vesicular route to the plasma membrane in cultured rat hepatocytes. *Gastroenterology* **108:** 1110–1123.

Roschlau G (1983) Hepatitis mit konfluierenden Nekrosen durch Dihydralazin (Depressan) *Zentalblatt für Allgemeine Pathologie und Anatomie* **127:** 385–393.

Roschlau G (1986) Virushepatitis gegen Arzneimittelhepatitis. *Zeitschrift für Klinische Medizin* **41:** 817–819.

Roy Chowdhury J, Wolkoff AW, Arias IM et al (1989) Inherited jaundice and disorders of bilirubin metabolism. In Scriver CR, Beaudet AL, Sly WS & Valle D (eds), *The Metabolic Basis of Inherited Disease*, 6th edn, pp 1085–1094. New York: Mc Graw-Hill.

Sacher M, Blumel P, Thaler H & Manns M (1990) Chronic active hepatitis associated with vitiligo, nail dystrophy, alopecia and a new variant of LKM antibodies. *Journal of Hepatology* **10:** 364–369.

Schröder LW, Siegmund W, Schneider T et al (1986) Zur Blutdruckwirksamkeit ausgewähler Dihydralazinmetabolite. *Pharmazie* **41:** 439.

Scully LJ, Toze C, Sengar DPS & Goldstein R (1993) Early-onset autoimmune hepatitis is associated with a C4A gene deletion. *Gastroenterology* **104:** 1478–1484.

Seki T, Kiyosawa K, Inoko H & Ota M (1990) Association of autoimmune hepatitis with HLA-Bw54 and DR4 in Japanese patients. *Hepatology* **12:** 1300–1304.

Siegmund W, Franke G, Biebler et al (1985) The influence of the acetylator phenotype on the clinical use of dihydralazine. *International Journal of Clinical Pharmacology and Therapeutic Toxicology* **23:** S74–S78.

Sipes IG, Gandolfi J, Pohl LR et al (1980) Comparision of the biotransformation and hepatotoxicity of halothane and deuterated halothane *Journal of Experimental Therapy* **214:** 716–720.

Sindelar WF, Tralka TS & Gibbs PS (1982) Evidence for acute cellular changes in human hepatocytes during anaesthesia with halohgenated agents: an electron microscopic study. *Surgery* **92:** 520–527.

Skoda RC, Gonzalez FJ, Derrierre A & Meyer UA (1988) Two mutant alleles of the human P450 db1 gene (P450C2D1) associated with genetically deficient metabolism of debrisoquine and other drugs. *Proceedings of the National Academy of Sciences of the USA* **85:** 5240–5243.

Smith GC, Kenna JG, Harrison DJ et al (1993) autoantibodies to hepatic microsomal carboxylesterase in halothane hepatitis. *Lancet* **342:** 963–964.

Song YH, Connor EL, Muir A et al (1994) Autoantibody epitope mapping in autoimmune Addison's Disease. *Journal of Clinical Endocrinology and Metabolism* **78:** 1108–1112.

Stacieki P & Oesch F (1980) Distribution of enzymes involved in metabolism of polycyclic aromatic hydrocarbons among rat liver endomembranes and plasma membranes. *European Journal of Cell Biology* **21:** 79–92.

Straub P, Philipp T, Lamb JG et al (1994) Molecular characterization of a microsomal antigen in hepatitis D. 45th Annual Meeting of the American Association for the Study of Liver Diseases. *Hepatology* **20:** 427.

Stricker BHC (1992) *Drug-Induced Hepatic Injury* Amsterdam: Elsevier.

Tait B, Mackay IR, Board PH et al (1989) HLA-AL -B8, -DR3 extended haplotypes in autoimmune chronic hepatitis. *Gastroenterology* **97:** 479–481.

Thomassen D, Martin BM, Martin JL et al (1989) The role of a stress protein in the development of drug induced allergic response. *European Journal of Pharmacology* **183:** 1138–1139.

Thomsen MS, Loft S, Roberts DW & Poulsen HE (1995) Cytochrome P450 2E1 inhibition by propylene glycol prevents acetaminophen (paracetamol) hepatotoxicizy in mice without cytochrome P450 1A2 inhibition. *Pharmacology and Toxicology* **76:** 395–399.

Tran A, Quaranta JF, Benzaken S et al (1993) High prevalence of thyrois antibodies in a prospective series of patients with chronic hepatitis C. *Hepatology* **18:** 253–257.

Trautwein C, Ramadori G, Gerken G et al (1992) Regulation of cytochrome P450 2D by acute phase mediators in C3H/HeJ mice. *Biochemical and Biophysical Research Communications* **182:** 617–623.

Trautwein C, Gerken G, Meyer zum Büschenfelde KH & Manns MP (1993) Lack of surface expression for the B-cell autoepitope of cytochrome P450 2D6 evidenced by flow cytometry. *Zeitschrift für Gastroenterologie* **31:** 225–230.

Trowell J, Peto R & Crampton Smith A (1975) Controlled trial of repeated halothane anaesthetics in patients with carcinoma of the uterine cervix treated with radium. *Lancet* **i:** 821–824.

Trudell JR, Ardies CM & Anderson WR (1991) Antibodies raised against trifluoroacetyl-protein adducts bind to N-trifluoroacetyl-phosphatidylethanolamine in hexagonal phase phospholipid micelles. *Journal of Pharmacological and Experimental Therapy* **257:** 657–662.

Uibo R, Aavik E, Peterson P et al (1994a) Autoantibodies to cytochrome P450 enzymes P450 see, P450 c17 and P450 c21 in Autoimmune Polyglandular Diseases types I and II and in isolated Addison's disease. *Journal of Clinical Endocrinology and Metabolism* **78:** 323–328.

Uibo R, Perheentupa J, Ovod V & Krohn KJE (1994b) Characterization of adrenal autoantigens recognized by serta from patients with autoimmune polyglandular syndrome (APS) type 1. *Journal of Autoimmunity* **7:** 399–411.

Van Pelt FN, Straub P & Manns MP(1995) Molecular basis of drug-induced immunological liver injury. *Seminars in Liver Disease* **15:** 283–300.

Vergani D, Wells L, Larcher VF et al (1985) Genetically determined low C4: a predisposing factor to autoimmune chronic active hepatitis. *Lancet* **ii:** 294–298.

Walton B, Simpson BR, Strunin L et al (1976) Unexplained hepatitis following halothane. *British Medical Journal* **1:** 1171–1176.

Winqvist O, Karlsson FA & Kämpe O (1992) 21-hydroxylase, a major autoantigen in idiopathic Addison's disease. *Lancet* **339:** 1559–1562.

Winqvist O, Gustafsson J, Rorsman F et al (1994) Two different cytochrome P450 enzymes are the adrenal antigens in autoimmune polyendocrine syndrome type 1 and addison's disease. *Journal of Clinical Investigation* **92:** 2377–2385

Winqvist O, Gebre-Mehedin G, Gustafsson et al (1995) Identification of the main gonadal autoantigens in patients with adrenal insufficiency and associated ovarian failure. *Journal of Clinical Endocrinology and Metabolism* **80:** 1717–1723.

Wittingham S, Mathews JD, Schanfield MS et al (1981) Interaction of HLA and Gm in autoimmune chronic active hepatitis. *Clinical and Experimental Immunology* **26:** 102–108.

Wright R, Eade OE, Chisolm M et al (1975) Controlled prospective study of the effect on liver function of multiple exposures to halothane. *Lancet* **i:** 817–820.

Wu D & Cederbaum AI (1992) Presence of functionally active cytochrome P4502E1 in the plasma membrane of rat hepatocytes. *Hepatology* **15:** 515–524.

Yamamoto AM, Mura C, De Lemos-Chiardini C et al (1993a) Cytochrome P450 2D6 recognized by LKM1 antibody is not expressed on the surface of hepatocytes. *Clinical and Experimental Immunology* **92:** 381–390.

Yamamoto AM, Cresteil D, Boniface O et al (1993b) Identification and analysis of cytochrome P450IID6 antigenic sites recognized by anti-liver-kidney microsome type-1 antibodies (LKM1) *European Journal of Immunology* **23:** 1105–1111.

Yamamoto AM, Crestil D, Homberg JC & Alvarez F (1993c) Characterization of anti-liver-kidney microsome antibodiy (anti-LKM1) from hepatitis C virus positive and negative sera. *Gastroenterology* **104:** 1762–1767.

Zanger UM, Hauri HP, Loeper J et al (1988) Antibodies against human cytochrome P450db1 in autoimmune hepatitis type II. *Proceedings of the National Academy of Sciences USA* **85:** 8256–8260.

Zimmerman HJ (1978) In Zimmerman HJ (ed.), *Hepatotoxiocity. The Adverse Effects of Drugs and Other Chemicals on the Liver*. New York: Appleton Century Crofts.

Zimmerman HJ, Lewis JH, Ishak KG & Maddrey W (1984) Ticrynafen-associated hepatic injury: analysis of 340 cases. *Hepatology* **4:** 315–323.

8

Immunogenetics in liver disease

PETER T. DONALDSON

Immunogenetics is concerned with studies of genes which regulate the immune response, and in particular with the polymorphic members of the 'immunoglobulin supergene family' (i.e. the genes of the major histocompatibility complex (MHC), the T cell receptor (TCR) and the immunoglobulin genes). Of these, the MHC is probably the most widely studied, with more than 70 genes spanning 4 million base-pairs of DNA in the distal portion of the 6p21.3 band on the short arm of chromosome 6. The classical MHC gene products are the human leukocyte antigens (HLAs) also referred to as transplantation or histocompatibility antigens.

Although the identification of HLA antigens was primarily associated with the development of clinical transplantation, early studies, dating from 1967, suggested that specific HLAs may be over-represented in some diseases. Furthermore, the degree to which these HLAs were associated with various diseases was found to be greater than that for any other genetic marker then known. Following these early discoveries there was enormous interest in HLA-encoded susceptibility/resistance to disease which reached a peak in the mid-1970s, and again in the mid-1980s following the discovery of the DR antigens (reviewed by Tiwari and Terasaki, 1985).

By the mid-to-late 1980s interest in HLA was beginning to wane because many of the associations described were weak and there was very limited understanding of the basic biology of HLA with its continuously changing nomenclature. Two publications, in the journal *Nature*, marked a change. The first was the description of X-ray crystallographic studies of the purified HLA molecule A2 (Bjorkman et al, 1987a,b) and the second was the association of specific amino acid residues of the HLA DQβ-polypeptide with susceptibility and resistance to insulin-dependent diabetes mellitus (IDDM) (Todd et al, 1987). These developments coupled with advances in molecular biology have led to a dramatic improvement in our understanding of HLA immunogenetics and mark the 'third age' for studies of HLA disease associations.

In this chapter I will review the evidence for HLA-encoded susceptibility to autoimmune and chronic viral liver diseases. Many of the early studies have been reviewed elsewhere (Donaldson et al, 1994; Manns and Kruger, 1994) and I will therefore concentrate on recent data, with particular emphasis on the molecular era.

Baillière's Clinical Gastroenterology—
Vol. 10, No. 3, September 1996
ISBN 0–7020–2187–3
0950–3528/96/030533 + 17 $12.00/00

GENETIC ORGANIZATION AND MOLECULAR STRUCTURE OF THE MHC PROTEINS

On the basis of biochemical, structural and functional studies, the MHC can be divided into three distinct regions referred to as HLA class I, HLA class II and HLA class III.

HLA class I

The HLA class I gene family has at least six functional genes coding for the cell-surface molecules HLA A, B, C, E, F and G and 12 pseudogenes (Geraghty, 1993). The HLA A, B and C molecules are constitutively expressed on most nucleated cells, although they are only weakly expressed or absent on endocrine cells, hepatocytes, smooth muscle, normal skeletal and cardiac muscle (Rose, 1993). In contrast HLA E, F and G have only limited tissue expression. The expressed HLA class I molecule is a hetero-dimer composed of a 45 kDa polypeptide (the α-chain) and a non-covalently bound 12 kDa β2-microglobulin molecule. The α-chain of the class I molecule exhibits extensive polymorphism. At present there are 59 recognized alleles of HLA-A, 119 of HLA-B and 36 of HLA-C, four of HLA-E and four of HLA-G (Bodmer et al, 1995). The β2-microglobulin molecule is a non-MHC gene product encoded on chromosome 15.

The α-chain spans the cell membrane and has three extra-cellular domains α1, α2 and α3. Different class I alleles result in amino acid substitutions primarily in the membrane distal α1 and α2 regions, while the membrane-proximal α3 region is relatively conserved between alleles (Bjorkman and Parham, 1990). X-ray crystallography of the class I molecule HLA-A2 shows the membrane-proximal domains of the molecule forming a 'stalk-like' structure which supports an eight-stranded anti-parallel β-pleated sheet surmounted by two α-helices (Bjorkman et al, 1987a,b). The β-pleated sheet and two α-helices form the floor and walls of a groove now known to be the site of antigen binding.

HLA class II—DR, DQ and DP

The HLA class II gene family includes a number of genes with diverse functions, including the classically described HLA class II molecules DR, DQ and DP, and also the genes for the TAP, LMP, DMA and DMB molecules (Campbell and Trowsdale, 1993). The classical class II HLAs are constitutively expressed on specialized antigen-presenting cells and may also be expressed on endothelial and epithelial cells (Rose, 1993).

The genetic organization of this region is complex (Campbell and Trowsdale, 1993). The DR region has a single DRA gene and nine DRB genes. Only four of the DRB genes *DRB1*, *DRB3*, *DRB4* and *DRB5* are expressed. All four are polymorphic. The remaining five DRB genes are pseudogenes. The number of expressed DRB molecules is dependent upon the *DRB1* allelic group, which is inherited as a discrete genetic unit or haplotype (Table 1). The HLA DQ and DP subregions each encode a single functional A gene (encoding the α-chain) and B gene (encoding the β-chain) and, in contrast to the DR genes, both DQA and DQB, DPA and DPB genes have extensive polymorphism. Presently there are two alleles of DRA, 138 alleles of the four expressed DRB genes, 24 alleles of DQA, 17 alleles of DQB, eight alleles of DPA and 62 alleles of DPB (Bodmer et al, 1995).

The expressed HLA class II molecule is a heterodimer composed of a 32 kDa α-chain which is non-covalently associated with a 28 kDa β-chain. Both the α- and β-polypeptides span the cell membrane, and each polypeptide chain has two extracellular domains. X-ray crystallography of the purified HLA class II molecule DR1 reveals secondary structure similar to that of the HLA class I molecule with an antigen-binding groove formed from the membrane distal α1 and β1 domains (Brown et al, 1993). As with HLA class I, different HLA class II alleles encode variations in the amino acid residues at specific positions in the antigen-binding groove (Kappes and Strominger, 1988; Gregersen, 1989).

Comparative analysis of the helical regions of the HLA class I and II grooves has revealed important structural differences. In the class I molecule the groove has relatively closed ends, favouring the binding of short peptides of nine amino acids or less. The class II groove is a much more open structure, allowing the linear binding of peptides of 12–24 amino acid residues which may project from either end. Specialized binding pockets have been recognized at polymorphic sites and these may anchor side-chains of the antigenic peptide, while the more conserved groove residues may interact with the main polypeptide chain (Madden, 1995; Rammensee, 1995)

Table 1. Organization of the HLA DRB genes in different haplotypes according to the DRB1 genomic group (genes in **bold** are pseudogenes).

DRB1 allelic group	Genomic organization				
*DRB1*01, DRB1*10*	DRB1	**DRB6**			**DRB9** DRA
*DRB1*15, DRB1*16*	DRB1	**DRB6** DRB5			**DRB9** DRA
*DRB1*03, DRB1*11* *DRB1*12, DRB1*13* *DRB1*14*	DRB1	**DRB2** DRB3			**DRB9** DRA
*DRB1*04, DRB1*07* *DRB1*09*	DRB1	**DRB7**	**DRB8**	DRB4	**DRB9** DRA
*DRB1*08*	DRB1				**DRB9** DRA

Non-classical HLA class II genes—TAP, LMP and DM

The class II region also includes a number of non-HLA genes. Of particular importance are the genes which encode proteins involved in processing antigen for presentation by HLA molecules. Peptide antigens destined to be presented at the cell surface by class I molecules are obtained from the cytoplasm (i.e. endogenous antigens) and are 'processed' into suitably sized, eight to nine amino acid peptides by interaction with a large multifunctional protease. The processed peptide then passes into the endoplasmic reticulum via a membrane associated transporter protein heterodimer, known as TAP (transporter associated with antigen processing). Two of the genes which may encode part of the large multifunctional protease (*LMP2* and *LMP7*) and the two genes encoding the TAP heterodimer (*TAP1* and *TAP2*) are located between the HLA DP and DQ loci. Of these genes LMP is thought to be non-polymorphic, but *TAP1* and *TAP2* show limited polymorphism, with five alleles of *TAP1* and four alleles of *TAP2*.

In contrast to class I molecules, which present endogenous antigen to CD8 T cells, class II molecules present exogenous antigen to CD4+ T cells. Class II molecules synthesized in the endoplasmic reticulum are prevented from binding to intra cellular peptides in the immediate vicinity by association with the invariant chain (Ii), a so-called 'molecular chaperone' (Williams and Watts, 1995). The stable class II heterodimer/ invariant chain complex migrates via the trans-Golgi to an acidic compartment (Schmid and Jackson, 1994). Here, a second molecule, also a heterodimer, DM, is thought to be involved in making the binding groove accessible for interaction with the antigenic peptides (Sloan et al, 1995). The DM locus is located between the DQ and DP genes and has both A and B genes each with four alleles.

HLA class III region

The genes of this region encode a diverse array of protein products but to date no cell-surface class III HLA heterodimers have been identified. Of particular interest are the polymorphic complement genes encoding the complement proteins C2, C4 (A and B) and factor B (Bf), and the genes for heat shock protein 70 (*HSP70*) and tumour necrosis factor α and β (*TNFA* and *TNFB*).

Nomenclature

The current WHO nomenclature is reviewed by Bodmer et al (1995). The nomenclature of those HLA determinants referred to in the text of this chapter is summarized in Table 2.

CLINICAL STUDIES

The general trend with HLA disease association studies has been to seek ever stronger associations, with 100% associations representing the 'holy grail'. However, such associations are rarely found. Many of the early studies were interpreted with the expectation that hidden close to the HLA genes on chromosome 6 were the actual *disease genes*. It is now generally realized that this is an unlikely explanation for these genetic associations, and more complex multifactorial/polygenic models are now being considered (Todd and Bain, 1992). In addition, early studies recognized that certain HLA antigens or alleles occur together more often than predicted

Table 2. Nomenclature for HLA antigens and genotypes used in this review.

Serological determinant		
Old name	Current Name	Allele[c]
HL-A1	A1	*A*0101, A*0102*
HL-A8	B8	*B*0801, B*0802*
	DR2	*DRB1*1501, DRB1*1502*
Dw3[a]	DR3[b]	*DRB1*03011, DRB1*03012*
Dw4[a]	DR4	*DRB1*0401*
Dw15[a]	DR4	*DRB1*0405*
DRw8	DR8	*DRB1*0801 to DRB1*0811*
DRw52a	DR52	*DRB3*0101*
DRw6	DR13	*DRB1*1301 to DRB1*1319*
DRw6	DR14	*DRB1*1401 to DRB1*1418*

[a] Denotes specificities determined by mixed lymphocyte reaction (MLR).
[b] The term DR17 or DRw17 has been used for common split of DR3 in caucasoid populations; however, this term was not widely used before it was replaced by the current WHO nomenclature.
[c] Current nomenclature is based on DNA sequencing data and is reviewed by Bodmer et al (1995).
The four-letter code denotes the locus, i.e. DRB1, the first two numbers following the asterisk represent the allelic group and are equivalent to the serologically defined antigen; thus, DRB1*03 = DR3, and the last two numbers represent the allele (based entirely on DNA sequencing data).

from the individual antigen frequencies. When this occurs the alleles are said to be in linkage disequilibrium. The best example of linkage disequilibrium is the HLA A1-B8-DR3 haplotype, present in 12–16% of Northern European populations, but if these genes were independently assorted these alleles should occur together in 2–3% of the population.

The methods used for HLA typing studies have evolved over the past decade with traditional serological methods and early DNA-based techniques giving way to more accurate methods based on polymerase chain reaction (PCR) amplification (reviewed by Donaldson et al, 1994).

Autoimmune liver diseases

While the pathological mechanisms remain unclear it is generally accepted that autoimmune hepatitis (AIH, sometimes called autoimmune chronic active hepatitis), primary sclerosing cholangitis (PSC) and primary biliary cirrhosis (PBC) are 'autoimmune' liver diseases, although only AIH fits the classical definition of Roitt (1971). Although family studies would offer a more powerful tool for elucidating the molecular genetics of these diseases, familial occurrences of AIH, PSC and PBC are exceedingly rare, and nearly all of the data we have come from population studies.

Autoimmune hepatitis

Early studies in AIH identified HLA A1, B8 and DR3 as susceptibility markers and indicated that the DR phenotype may correlate with the age of onset (reviewed by Donaldson et al, 1994; Manns and Kruger, 1994). There followed a decade of conflicting reports (Tiwari and Terasaki, 1985; Donaldson et al, 1991a). In 1991, a study of 96 AIH patients from King's College Hospital suggested that susceptibility to AIH was determined by HLA DR3 and DR4 and that these two class II antigens identified distinct subsets of the disease. One subset was the DR3-associated, early onset, severe form of AIH and the other was the DR4-associated, late onset, less severe form of the disease (Donaldson et al, 1991a). These data were supported by observations from Japan, where the characteristic age of onset of AIH correlates with that of the older-onset European AIH patients, and where 90.3% of AIH patients have DR4 (Seki et al, 1990).

These findings were further investigated using PCR genotyping by Doherty et al (1994a) with two objectives, first, to identify stronger associations with HLA DQA and DQB, and second, to seek a common determinant shared by those with DR3 and those with DR4-associated disease. As expected, the patients had a very high frequency of the HLA *DRB1*0301-DRB3*0101-DQA1*0501-DQB1*0201* haplotype (52% versus 19% of controls), and there was a strong secondary association with one of the DR4 alleles *DRB1*0401* (54% of *DRB3*0101*-negative patients compared to 23.3% of *DRB3*0101*-negative controls). The data suggested that the DRB genes were more strongly associated with the disease than either DQA or DQB. In pursuing the second objective in Doherty's study, it was found that a single amino acid residue, lysine, at position 71 of the HLA DRβ-polypeptide (which is encoded by *DRB1*0301* and *DRB1*0401* and also by all of the *DRB3* alleles), was present in 94% of patients compared to 64% controls. However, in Japan the predominant DR4 subtype in AIH is *DRB1*0405*, which does not encode a lysine residue at DRβ71 (Ota et al, 1992). Two mutually exclusive hypotheses were published, one based on lysine at DRβ71 (Doherty et al, 1994a), and the second based on basic amino acids at DRβ13 (Ota et al, 1992). A second, independent series of 86 caucasoid AIH patients from the Mayo Clinic has recently been investigated in our laboratory and the analysis, although preliminary, confirms the lysine DRβ71 hypothesis (Strettell et al, 1996).

The idea that the basis of immunogenetic susceptibility to AIH in Northern Europe is different to that seen in Japan is not surprising as the two populations are genetically dissimilar. However, the reports from Argentina of HLA genotypes in paediatric AIH patients (Fainboim et al, 1994) and adult AIH patients (Marcos et al, 1994) also appear to contradict the lysine DRβ71 hypothesis. In these reports, *DRB1*1301*, which does not encode lysine at DRβ71, appears to be the primary susceptibility allele for early-onset AIH and DR4 for late-onset AIH. This is a very significant variation from the Northern European and North American data and there is no good reason why these genetic associations should differ as both populations have a similar ethnic background. It is possible that the primary susceptibility allele for early-onset AIH in Argentinean patients is encoded by the other expressed DRB gene carried on the *DRB1*1301* haplotype, i.e. the *DRB3* genes, all of which encode lysine at β71. Although the latter hypothesis was discounted by Fainboim et al (1994) it has not been rigorously tested.

The associations described above in Argentinean patients highlight two points of interest. First, that there are different HLA associations for adult and paediatric patients, perhaps representing different forms of the disease, or more severe forms of the disease. In our own series DR4 was present in only two out of 38 (5%) children with AIH compared to an expected frequency of 39% (Germana et al (1996), manuscript submitted for publication). In adult patients from King's and the Mayo Clinic, those with B8 or DR3 presented earlier and were more likely to relapse while on treatment (Czaja et al, 1990, Donaldson et al; 1991a). In contrast, recent data suggest that those with DR4 are more likely to have concurrent extrahepatic disease (Marcos et al, 1994; Czaja et al (1996), manuscript submitted for publication). Even in the study of Doherty et al, (1994a), although there is a common susceptibility determinant (lysine β71), those with *DRB1*0301*, had more severe disease than those with *DRB1*0401*, suggesting that other genes may determine severity and age of onset. One possibility is that this is caused by the number of lysine-DRβ71 residues (i.e. a gene-dosage effect). In those with *DRB1*0301*, the second expressed DRB gene, *DRB3*0101*, also carries a lysine residue at DRβ71 whereas in those with *DRB1*0401* the second expressed DRB gene, DRB4*0103, does not (Strettell et al, 1995).

The other major candidates both as susceptibility genes and as a determinants of disease severity are the HLA class III complement genes. Persistently low levels of C4 are a common feature of AIH and are associated with deleted and non-expressed *C4A* and *C4B* genes (Vergani et al, 1985; Scully et al, 1993; Doherty et al, 1994b). Analysis of the contribution that complement genes make to susceptibility to AIH is complicated by the fact that the *C4A* null gene is in strong linkage disequilibrium with the A1-B8-DR3-DQ2 haplotype. However it is worth noting that *C4B* null genes co-segregate with HLA DR4 and therefore C4 genes may be important in both A1-B8-DR3-encoded and DR4-encoded susceptibility to AIH.

Primary sclerosing cholangitis

Immunogenetic studies of PSC date from 1982 and 1983 when B8 and DR3 were reported as susceptibility factors in three small studies (reviewed by Donaldson et al, 1994). Following these reports there was a decade of silence until, in the early 1990s, two studies based on HLA serotyping precipitated sufficient interest for a molecular re-evaluation of HLA-encoded susceptibility to PSC. The first study of 81 PSC patients confirmed existing associations with B8 and DR3 (Donaldson et al, 1991b), suggested that the susceptibility lies closer to DR than to the HLA A or B loci, and identified a new association with HLA DR2 in patients with late-onset disease. This dual association may be the result of linkage with a susceptibility allele shared by DR2 and DR3 or, alternatively, may define distinct subsets of PSC. The second landmark study by Prochazka et al (1990) reported DRw52a in 29 out of 29 (100%) patients. Initially this report generated great excitement; however, subsequent correspondence (Olerup et al (1991) *New England Journal of Medicine* **325:** 1252 (correspondence);

Mehal et al (1991) *New England Journal of Medicine* **325:** 1252 (correspondence)) refuted the findings, which were later withdrawn (Park et al (1991) *New England Journal of Medicine* **325:** 1252). Despite this, Prochazka's study was instrumental in focusing attention on the DR52a allele (correctly named *DRB3*0101*) which is encoded by the *DRB3* gene and is present on most DR3 haplotypes, especially the A1-B8-DR3 haplotype.

The first extensive molecular evaluation of HLA-encoded susceptibility in PSC was undertaken by Farrant et al (1992). The study was designed to identify possible new associations at the HLA DQA and DQB loci and detect a common determinant shared by those with DR2 and those with DR3-associated disease. As expected, the patients had a very high frequency of the *HLA DRB1*0301-DRB3*0101-DQA1*0501-DQB1*0201* haplotype (39% versus 19% of controls) but the study did not confirm the association with DR2. In addition, a new association with the *DRB1*1301-DRB3*0101-DQA1*0103-DQB1*0603* haplotype and negative association with the *DRB1*0401* allele were described. The data suggested that the DRB genes were more strongly associated with the disease than either DQA or DQB, an observation which was supported by DPB genotyping of the same series (Underhill et al 1995). Since both *DRB1*0301* and *DRB1*1301* are in linkage disequilibrium with *DRB3*0101* (DR52a), it was suggested that *DRB3*0101* may be the primary susceptibility allele in PSC. Further analysis suggested that the previous report of a secondary association with DR2 in DR3-negative patients may result from linkage disequilibrium with *DRB5*0101*. The alleles *DRB3*0101* and *DRB5*0101* were present in 79% of patients in Farrant's series and since both alleles encode a leucine residue at position 38 of the DRβ polypeptide, while all other DRB alleles encode alanine or valine at β38, a model of susceptibility based on leucine β38 was proposed.

The basic observations from this study were confirmed in two later studies, the Oxford group showed that susceptibility to PSC is determined by HLA *DRB1*0301* and *DRB3*0101* (Mehal et al 1994a) and a second study from Sweden confirmed the associations with *DRB1*0301*, *DRB3*0101* and the *DRB1*1301-DQA1*0103-DQB1*0603* haplotype (Olerup et al 1995). Furthermore, in both studies there was a reduced frequency of *DRB1*04* in patients compared to controls. However, although these two studies confirmed the underlying HLA associations in PSC there is considerable controversy over the interpretation of the data, particularly in respect to the identity of the primary susceptibility allele, the leucine β38 model and the role of DR4 in determining prognosis. While the two UK studies agreed that *DRB3*0101* is the primary susceptibility allele, Olerup et al (1995) argued that this is secondary to the associations with *DRB1*0301* and *DRB1*1301*. In addition, the leucine β38 model is undermined by the observation that the association with leucine β38 was weaker than for *DRB3*0101* in the Swedish series, the major difference between the studies resulting from the finding of a similar frequency of the *DRB5*0101* allele in Swedish patients and controls. The third controversy is one of greater clinical importance, and surrounds the observation from

Oxford that DR4 is a marker of rapid disease progression in PSC (Mehal et al 1994a). This observation appears to be contrary (although it is not necessarily so) to the observation of a negative association with DR4 in PSC which was found in all three studies and would usually be interpreted as conferring protection from the disease. Neither our own unpublished data (Donaldson, unpublished observations, 1996) nor the Swedish series have confirmed Mehal's hypothesis.

Primary biliary cirrhosis (PBC)

Of the numerous early studies describing HLA associations in PBC, only the association with DR8 (Gores et al, 1987) has been confirmed (Underhill et al, 1992; Gregory et al 1993; Begovich et al 1994). However, the association with DR8 in European and American white populations is weak, accounting for only 11–36% of patients studied. This may be an indication that the 'susceptibility allele' in PBC lies some distance from the HLA DR genes. The primary susceptibility allele is unlikely to be either DQB or DPB because the only DQB association described in PBC, with the *DQB1*0402* allele, appears to be due to linkage with DR8 (Underhill et al, 1992; Begovich et al, 1994) and, to date, there are no reported associations with the HLA DPB alleles in Europe (Underhill et al, 1995) or North America (Begovich et al, 1994). Two HLA class III complement genes have been identified as possible susceptibility alleles *C4B2* (Briggs et al, 1987; Mehal et al, 1994b) and *C4AQ0* (Manns et al, 1991). It has been proposed that both *C4B2* and *C4AQ0* are in linkage disequilibrium with DR8 in PBC, although this is in contrast to the expected pattern of linkage disequilibrium for C4 and DR alleles in Europeans (Baur et al, 1984).

More recently, Begovich et al (1994) suggested that the *DQA1*0102* allele confers resistance to PBC, having found reduced frequencies of the *DRB1*1501-DQA1*0102-DQB1*0602* and *DRB1*1302-DQA1*0102-DQB1*0604* haplotypes, both of which include the *DQA1*0102* allele. Although the latter observations require independent confirmation, in our own studies, which used RFLP analysis for DRB assignments, the frequency of *DRB1*15* was marginally reduced being present in 33/159 (21%) of patients compared to 46/162 (29%) of controls, and there were also similar trends for *DQB1*0602* and *DQB1*0604* (Underhill et al, 1992). Unfortunately, *DQA1* genotypes were not evaluated in our series. In addition in the series by Gregory et al (1993) there was a lower frequency of DR13 in patients compared to controls (15/130, 11.5% versus 67/363, 18.4%).

Much stronger HLA associations with PBC have been reported from Japan, where between 36.8% and 78.6% of patients are DR8-positive (Maeda et al, 1992; Seki et al, 1993) and the DR8 haplotype most commonly seen in PBC is *DRB1*08-DQB1*03-DPB1*0501* (Seki et al 1993) with up to 85% of patients being *DPB1*0501*-positive. On the basis of these data, Seki et al (1993) proposed that *DPB1*0501* may be the primary susceptibility allele for PBC in Japan and, when further analysis revealed that 43 of the 47 Japanese patients (91.4%) have a leucine residue at position 35 of the DPβ polypeptide, the authors proposed that leucine at DPβ35 may be the basis of susceptibility to PBC in that population. Two recently published studies from Japan are at odds with Seki's hypothesis. Oguri et al (1994) proposed a model of susceptibility based on leucine at DRβ74, and Mukai et al (1995) found no significant increase in the *DPB1*0501* allele and suggested that the primary susceptibility allele for PBC in Japan is the *DRB1*0803* allele.

HLA and hepatitis virus infection

Hepatitis B virus infection

Early studies of HLA in patients with hepatitis B virus infection showed that there was no association with HLA A1 or B8, and reports of an association with B35 were unconfirmed (Tiwari and Terasaki, 1985). More recently, HLA and HBV infection has been re-examined, most notably in two studies. The first, using RFLP analysis, described a reduced frequency of DR2 and increased frequency of DR7 in 34 patients with chronic persistent HBV infection from Qatar (Almarri and Batchelor, 1994). The second described the protective effect of the DR6 allele *DRB1*1302* in 185 children with chronic persistent HBV infection from the Gambia (Thursz et al, 1995). DR7 has been linked with hypo-responsiveness to the HBV vaccine Hepatavax-B (Craven et al, 1986; Weisman and Tsuchiyose, 1988) and DR6 has been linked with viral clearance (van Hattum et al, 1987) and a favourable response to interferon therapy (Scully et al, 1990) in Northern European patients.

The close association which exists between hepatitis B virus and the development of hepatocellular carcinoma (HCC) has lead to the search for host genes which may modulate the effect of virus infection and increase the risk of HCC developing. Early reports of HLA and HCC reported no association but were mostly restricted to HLA class I alleles (Tiwari and Terasaki, 1985). More recently we have reported an extensive survey of HLA class II DRB, DQA, DQB and DPB alleles in Hong Kong Chinese patients with HCC, with and without HBV infection, and have similarly negative results (Johnson et al, 1996, manuscript submitted for publication).

Hepatitis C virus infection

The development of accurate diagnostic tests for the detection of hepatitis C virus is a relatively recent phenomenon and therefore there has been little chance to study the immunogenetics of this disease. The one published study found no association with HLA A, B serotype and DR RFLP patterns in 75 north American patients with chronic HCV infection, but did report that concurrent immunological disease is associated with HLA DR4 (Czaja et al, 1995). A recent (unpublished) study of 102 patients with chronic HCV infection from King's College Hospital found no association at HLA A, B or DR but a strong protective effect of the *DQA1*03* allele (Tibbs et al,

1996, manuscript submitted for publication). This contrasts with preliminary data from Marousis et al (1995), who reported an association with the *DQB1*05* alleles, and also conflicts with a number of earlier reports of HLA associations in so-called type II AIH patients many of whom were HCV positive (reviewed by Manns and Kruger, 1994).

DISCUSSION

There are two different interpretations we can use to explain these HLA associations: either the HLA molecule is directly involved in the development of the disease process (i.e. through antigen presentation) or these genes are markers of disease severity. Both possibilities will be discussed here.

Mechanisms of HLA encoded disease susceptibility

The strong HLA associations reviewed above (summarized in Table 3), suggest that these genes are not simply markers, by virtue of linkage disequilibrium, for an undiscovered *disease gene*. Indeed, linkage disequilibrium and the degree of heterogeneity in the definition of any specific disease where the pathological process is unknown bar the way to identifying closer genetic markers for AIH and possibly PSC, although not necessarily PBC or viral liver disease.

A number of possible mechanisms for autoimmunity exist, although not all can explain how HLA molecules may predispose to disease. One such theory is the molecular mimicry hypothesis (reviewed by Baum et al, 1996). Although the asialoglycoprotein receptor (ASGPR), a putative autoantigen in AIH, and PDC-E2 peptide, a putative autoantigen in PBC, both share sequence homology with the DRα-polypeptide, the DRA gene is not polymorphic. If this peptide acts as a molecular mimic in these two diseases then there must be an alternative explanantion for the HLA association reviewed above.

All autoimmune diseases involve some degree of failure of self tolerance. Complete self tolerance depends on the total absence of self-reactive T cells, and may be achieved either through deletion of self-reactive clones during thymic development (clonal deletion) or through the active suppression of T cells recognizing self-antigens (peripheral tolerance). It has been hypothesized that failure to induce tolerance is more likely to occur if there is weak binding of the self-peptide to class II molecules (Nepom, 1990; Sheehy, 1992). Class II molecules associated with an increased risk of a given disease may bind the autoantigenic peptide with low affinity, while those class II molecules which are associated with a reduced risk of disease may bind the autoantigenic peptide with high affinity.

From a molecular view point, HLA gene polymorphisms, which result in different amino acid residues along the α-helical regions and the floor of

Table 3. Key HLA associations with autoimmune and chronic viral liver disease.

Disease	Key haplotype or allele	Population[a]	Effect
AIH	A*01..-B*08..-**DRB3*0101-DRB1*0301-DQA1*0501-DQB1*0201**[b]	Caucasoid	Susceptibility
	...........-DRB4*0103-**DRB1*0401**	Caucasoid	Susceptibility
	...........-DRB4*...-**DRB1*0405**....................	Japanese	Susceptibility
	...........-B*07..-**DRB5*0101-DRB1*1501**-DQA1*0102-DQB1*0602	Caucasoid	Resistance
PSC	A*01..-B*08..-**DRB3*0101-DRB1*0301**-DQA1*0501-DQB1*0201[c]	Caucasoid	Susceptibility
	...........-**DRB3*0101-DRB1*1301**-DQA1*0103-DQB1*0603	Caucasoid	Susceptibility
	...........-DRB4*0103-**DRB1*0401**....................	Caucasoid	Resistance
PBC	...........DRB1*0801-DQA1*0401-DQB1*0402.............	Caucasoid	Susceptibility
	...........**DRB1*0803-DQA1*...-DQB1*03..-DPB1*0501**[c]	Japanese	Susceptibility
	...........-DRB5*0101-DRB1*1501-**DQA1*0102-DQB1*0602**[d]	Caucasoid	Resistance
	...........-DRB3*...-DRB1*1302-**DQA1*0102-DQB1*0604**[d]	Caucasoid	Resistance
Chronic HBV	....................**DRB1*1302**[d]........................	Gambia	Resistance
Chronic HCV	...........-DRB4*....-DRB1*04..-**DQA1*03**[d]	Caucasoid	Resistance

Where there are incomplete genotypes the alleles at these loci have not been tested or are not associated with the disease (see text). The alleles in bold are those which are thought to be the key elements in each haplotype.

[a] The caucasoids association are based on studies on North American and European populations and on those of European origin.

[b] Current data strongly suggest that DRB1 is the key gene in AIH (Strettell et al, 1996).

[c] The key element in these haplotypes is currently controversial (see text).

[d] These associations are yet to be confirmed in independent series.

the antigen-binding groove, may dramatically affect the conformation and orientation with which the peptide is bound and presented to the TCR. These variations in the amino acid sequences will not only affect the recognition of the peptide by the TCR, but also the interaction between the TCR and the HLA molecule. Furthermore, different HLA alleles may encode HLA molecules with differing affinities for antigenic peptides. It is possible that a hierarchy of self-peptide binding by susceptible and protective class II alleles is the basis of autoimmunity. Thus, an HLA DR molecule bearing a lysine residue at position β71, or leucine at β38 and an HLA DP molecule bearing a leucine residue at position 35 of the DPβ-polypeptide may have low binding affinity for self-peptides thereby rendering an individual susceptible to AIH or PSC or PBC either through failure of clonal deletion or via failure of peripheral tolerance.

A similar hypothesis may account for HLA associations with infectious diseases; thus, low-affinity binding of viral peptides may result in poor viral clearance and facilitate chronic infection, while high-affinity binding may lead to efficient viral clearance and protect the host from chronic infection. This may account for the protective effect of the *DRB1*1302* allele in HBV infection in the Gambia (Thursz et al, 1995) and also the effect of the *DQB1*05* and *DQA1*03* alleles in chronic HCV infection (Marousis et al, 1995; Tibbs et al, 1996, manuscript submitted for publication). The high prevalence and conserved nature of some HLA haplotypes, especially A1-B8-DR3, suggests that these genes confer some selective advantage upon a population despite the almost ubiquitous association with autoimmune disease. It has been suggested that susceptibility to autoimmune disease may be the penalty acquired by a population for increased resistance to infectious diseases (Benacerraf, 1981; de Vries, 1992; Hill et al, 1991; Thursz et al, 1995). Clearly, more work needs to be done to define these susceptibility alleles, especially in relation to chronic viral liver diseases.

HLA and severity of disease

The hypothesis that HLA associations are simply markers of more rapid disease progression and severity of symptoms is supported by the finding of an association of DR4 with late-onset AIH and the observation that AIH and PSC patients with A1-B8-DR3 present earlier in life and relapse more frequently while receiving conventional therapies (Czaja et al, 1990; Donaldson et al, 1991a,b; Farrant et al, 1992; Doherty et al, 1994a). This does not belittle the importance of HLA disease associations but may alter their interpretation and may explain the differing results reported from various centres.

DIRECTIONS FOR FUTURE STUDIES

In Northern European patients with AIH and PSC the DRB locus appears to encode the primary susceptibility alleles. However, not all patients are accounted for by the models reviewed above, and the predominance of the extended A1-B8-DR3 haplotype as a susceptibility marker in AIH, PSC and most other autoimmune diseases may indicate the presence of more than one susceptibility gene on this haplotype (Todd J., personal communication, March, 1995). It is also possible that the products of the class II genes interact to form novel α/β heterodimers (Lotteau et al, 1987). The *trans* pairing of DQα and DQβ-chains encoded on different haplotypes has been identified as a susceptibility factor for IDDM (Nepom et al, 1987; Ronningen et al, 1991).

Finally, it is likely that there may be several genes, both within and outside the MHC region that encode susceptibility to these diseases. Recent studies of IDDM suggest that there may be as many as 18 susceptibility alleles (Todd and Bain, 1992). One or more of these genes may contribute to a permissive environment for the generation of IDDM. Similarly, in autoimmune liver disease several genes may act, either individually or in concert, as a permissive gene pool for the generation of liver damage. A number of other MHC and non-MHC genes should be investigated as candidate susceptibility loci, including HLA Cw, the HLA class III region genes, TAP, LMP and DM and non-MHC genes involved in peptide recognition such as the T-cell receptor and the immunoglobulin genes. In addition, for each of these genes, polymorphism of the upstream promoters and regulatory transcription factors should also be considered.

SUMMARY

Recent advances in molecular biology, in particular X-ray crystallography of the purified antigens A2 and DR1 and development of PCR-based HLA genotyping techniques, has revolutionized our understanding of immunogenetics and cellular immunology. The application of molecular immunogenetics has refined our understanding of HLA-encoded susceptibility and resistance to both autoimmune and chronic viral liver disease. Recent studies of autoimmune hepatitis (AIH), primary sclerosing cholangitis (PSC) and primary biliary cirrhosis (PBC) have identified substitutions of specific amino acid residues in the HLA DRβ-polypeptide (AIH and PSC) and DPβ-polypeptide (PBC) which may determine susceptibility to and resistance from disease. Although these models of HLA-encoded susceptibility in PSC and PBC are currently controversial, the model for AIH, based on lysine residue at DRβ71 has recently been confirmed in an independent series. Data on chronic viral liver disease are less abundant, but a number of interesting observations are beginning to emerge. In the Gambia, resistance to chronic hepatitis B infection has been associated with the HLA *DRB1*1302* allele, and in studies of patients with chronic hepatitis C virus infection *DQA1*03* and *DQB1*05* have been identified as a possible protective factors.

Clarifying these HLA associations is not simply an academic pursuit; in addition to providing useful clues to the pathogenesis of these diseases, HLA associations may be important indicators of prognosis. In AIH, patients with the *DRB1*0301-DRB3*0101* haplotype appear to have more severe disease than those with *DRB1*0401*, while in PSC, *DRB3*0101* is associated with early onset of disease and *DRB1*0401* may be a marker of more rapid disease progression. To date, our knowledge of immunogenetic susceptibility in liver disease is incomplete and further work is needed.

REFERENCES

Almarri A & Batchelor JR (1994) HLA and hepatitis B infection. *Lancet* **344:** 1194–1195.

Baum H, Davies H & Peakman M (1996) Molecular mimicry in the MHC: hidden clues to auto-immunity? *Immunology Today* **17:** 64–70.

Baur MP, Neugebauer M & Albert ED (1984) Reference table of two-locus haplotype frequencies for all MHC marker loci. In Albert ED, Baur MP & Mayr WR (eds) *Histocompatibility Testing,* pp 667–755. New York: Springer Verlag.

Begovich AB, Klitz W, Moonsamy PV et al (1994) Genes within the HLA class II region confer pre-disposition and resistance to primary biliary cirrhosis. *Tissue Antigens* **43:** 71–77.

Benacerraf B (1981) Role of MHC gene products in immune regulation. *Science* **212:** 1229–1238.

Bjorkman PJ & Parham P (1990) Structure, function, and diversity of class I major histocompatibil-ity complex molecules. *Annual Review of Biochemistry* **59:** 253–288.

Bjorkman PJ, Saper MA, Samraoui B et al (1987a) Structure of human class I histocompatibility antigen, HLA-A2. *Nature* **329:** 506–512.

Bjorkman PJ, Saper MA, Samraoui B et al (1987b) The foreign antigen binding site and T cell recognition regions of class I histocompatibility antigens. *Nature* **329:** 512–518.

Bodmer JG, Marsh SGE, Albert ED et al (1995) Nomenclature for factors of the HLA system, 1995. *Tissue Antigens* **46:** 1–18.

Briggs DC, Donaldson PT, Hayes P et al (1987) A major histocompatibility complex Class III allo-type *C4B2* associated with primary biliary cirrhosis. *Tissue Antigens* **29:** 141–145.

Brown JH, Jardetzky TS, Gorga JC et al (1993) Three-dimensional structure of the human class II histocompatibility antigen HLA-DR1. *Nature* **364:** 33–39.

Campbell RD & Trowsdale J (1993) Map of the human MHC. *Immunology Today* **14:** 349–352.

Craven DE, Awdeh ZL & Kunches LM (1986) Non responsiveness to hepatitis B vaccine in health care workers. *Annals of Internal Medicine* **105:** 356–360.

Czaja AJ, Rakela J, Hay JE et al (1990) Clinical and prognostic implications of HLA B8 in cortico-steroid-treated severe autoimmune chronic active hepatitis. *Gastroenterology* **98:** 1587–1593.

Czaja AJ, Carpenter HA, Santrach PJ & Breanndan-Moore S (1995) Immunological features and HLA associations in chronic viral hepatitis. *Gastroenterology* **108:** 157–164.

de Vries RRP (1992) HLA and disease: from epidemiology to immunotherapy. *European Journal of Clinical Investigation* **22:** 1–8.

Doherty DG, Donaldson PT, Underhill JA et al (1994a) Allelic sequence variation in the HLA class II genes and proteins in patients with autoimmune hepatitis. *Hepatology* **19:** 609–615.

Doherty DG, Underhill JA, Donaldson PT et al (1994b). Polymorphism in the human complement C4 genes and susceptibility to autoimmune hepatitis. *Autoimmunity* **18:** 243–249.

Donaldson PT, Doherty DG, Hayllar KM et al (1991a) Susceptibility to autoimmune chronic active hepatitis: human leucocyte antigens DR4 and A1-B8-DR3 are independent risk factors. *Hepatology* **13:** 701–706.

Donaldson PT, Farrant JM, Wilkinson ML et al (1991b). Dual association of HLA DR2 and DR3 with primary sclerosing cholangitis. *Hepatology* **13:** 129–133.

Donaldson P, Doherty D, Underhill J & Williams R (1994) The molecular genetics of autoimmune liver disease. *Hepatology* **20:** 225–239.

Fainboim L, Marcos Y, Pando M et al (1994) Chronic active autoimmune hepatitis in children: strong association with a particular HLA-DR6 (*DRB1*1301*) haplotype. *Human Immunology* **41:** 146–150.

Farrant JM, Doherty DG, Donaldson PT et al (1992) Amino acid substitutions at position 38 of the DRβ polypeptide confer susceptibility and protection from primary sclerosing cholangitis. *Hepatology* **16:** 390–395.

Geraghty DE (1993) Structure of the HLA class I region and expression of its resident genes. *Current Opinion in Immunology* **5:** 3–7.

Gores GJ, Moore SB, Fisher LD et al (1987) Primary biliary cirrhosis: association with class II major histocompatibility complex antigens. *Hepatology* **7**: 889–892.

Gregersen PK (1989) Biology of disease: HLA class II polymorphism: implications for susceptibility to autoimmune disease. *Laboratory Investigation* **61**: 5–19.

Gregory W, Mehal W, Dunn AN et al (1993) Primary biliary cirrhosis: contribution of HLA class II allele DR8. *Quarterly Journal of Medicine* **86**: 393–399.

Hill AVS, Allsopp CEM, Kwiatkowski D et al (1991) Common West African HLA antigens are associated with protection from severe malaria. *Nature* **352**: 595–600.

Kappes D & Strominger JL (1988) Human class II major histocompatibility complex genes and proteins. *Annual Review of Biochemistry* **57**: 991–1028.

Lotteau V, Teyton L, Burroughs D et al (1987) A novel HLA class II molecule (DRα-DQβ) created by mismatched isotype pairing. *Nature* **329**: 339–341.

Madden DR (1995) The three-dimensional structure of peptide-MHC complexes. *Annual Review of Immunology* **13**: 587–622.

Maeda T, Onoshi S, Saibara T et al (1992) HLA DR8 and primary biliary cirrhosis. *Gastroenterology* **103**: 1118–1119.

Manns M & Kruger M (1994) Immunogenetics of chronic liver disease. *Gastroenterology* **106**: 1676–1697.

Manns MP, Bremm A, Schneider PM et al (1991) HLA DRw8 and complement C4 deficiency as risk factors in primary biliary cirrhosis. *Gastroenterology* **101**: 1367–1373.

Marcos Y, Fainboim HA, Capucchio M et al (1994) Two-locus involvement in the association of human leukocyte antigen with the extrahepatic manifestations of autoimmune chronic active hepatitis. *Hepatology* **19**: 1371–1374.

Marousis CG, She JX, She JY et al (1995) Differential prevalence of HLA class II DQB1 but not DRB1 alleles in Caucasian patients with chronic hepatitis C. Abstracts of the American Association for the Study of the Liver. *Hepatology* **22**: 349A.

Mehal WZ, Lo Y-M D, Wordsworth BP et al (1994a) HLA DR4 is a marker for rapid disease progression in primary sclerosing cholangitis. *Gastroenterology* **106**: 160–167.

Mehal WZ, Gregory WL, Lo D et al (1994b) Defining the immunogenetic susceptibility to primary biliary cirrhosis. *Hepatology* **20**: 1213–1219.

Mukai T, Kimura A, Ishibashi H et al (1995) Association of *HLA-DRB1 *0803* and *1602* with susceptibility to primary biliary cirrhosis. *International Hepatology Communications* **3**: 207–212.

Nepom GT (1990) A unified hypothesis for the complex genetics of HLA associations with IDDM. *Diabetes* **39**: 1153–1157.

Nepom BS, Schwartz D, Palmer JP et al (1987) Transcomplementation of HLA genes in IDDM. HLA-DQ α- and β-chains produce hybrid molecules in DR3/DR4 heterozygotes. *Diabetes* **36**: 114–117.

Oguri H, Oba S, Ogina H et al (1994) Susceptibility to primary biliary cirrhosis is associated with human leukocyte antigen *DRB1*0803* in Japanese patients. *International Hepatology Communications* **2**: 263–270.

Olerup O, Olsson R, Hultcrantz R et al (1995) HLA-DR and HLA-DQ are not markers for rapid disease progression in primary sclerosing cholangitis. *Gastroenterology* **108**: 870–878.

Ota M, Seki T, Kiyosawa K et al (1992) A possible association between basic amino acids at position 13 of *DRB1* chains and autoimmune hepatitis. *Immunogenetics* **36**: 49–55.

Prochazka EJ, Terasaki PI, Park MS et al (1990) Association of primary sclerosing cholangitis with HLA DRw52a. *New England Journal of Medicine* **322**: 1842–1844.

Rammensee H-G (1995) Chemistry of peptides associated with MHC class I and class II molecules. *Current Opinion in Immunology* **7**: 85–96.

Roitt IM (1971) *Essential Immunology*. Oxford: Blackwell Scientific Publications.

Ronningen KS, Gjertsen HA, Iwe T et al (1991) Particular HLA DQ αβ heterodimer associated with IDDM susceptibility in both DR4-DQw4 Japanese and DR4-DQw8/DRw8-DQw4 whites. *Diabetes* **40**: 759–763.

Rose ML (1993) HLA antigens in tissues. In Dyer P & Middleton D (eds) *Histocompatibility Testing*, pp 191–210. Oxford: Oxford University Press.

Schmid SL & Jackson MR (1994) Making class II presentable. *Nature* **369**: 103–104.

Scully L, Brown D, Lloyd C et al (1990) Immunological studies before and during interferon therapy in chronic HBV infection: identification of factors predicting response. *Hepatology* **12**: 1111–1117.

Scully LJ, Toze C, Sengar DPS et al (1993) Early-onset autoimmune hepatitis is associated with a C4A gene deletion. *Gastroenterology* **104:** 1478–1484.

Seki T, Kiyosawa K, Inoko H et al (1990) Association of autoimmune hepatitis with HLA-Bw54 and DR4 in Japanese patients. *Hepatology* **12:** 1300–1304.

Seki T, Kiyosawa K, Ota M et al (1993) Association of primary biliary cirrhosis with human leucocyte antigen *DPB1*0501* in Japanese patients. *Hepatology* **18:** 73–78.

Sheehy MJ (1992) HLA and insulin-dependent diabetes. A protective perspective. *Diabetes* **41:** 123–129.

Sloan VS, Cameron P, Porter G et al (1995) Mediation by HLA-DM of dissociation of peptides from HLA-DR. *Nature* **375:** 802–806.

Strettell MDJ, Czaja A, Donaldson PT & Williams R (1995) Genetic susceptibility to autoimmune hepatitis. Abstracts of the American Association for the Study of the Liver, *Hepatology* **22:** 128A.

Strettell MDJ, Czaja A, Thomson LJ et al (1996) Susceptibility to autoimmune hepatitis (AIH) is determined by a lysine residue at position 71 of the DRβ polypeptide chain. Abstracts of the American Gastroenterological Association. *Gastroenterology* **110:** A1335.

Thursz MR, Kwiatkowski D, Allsopp CEM et al (1995) Association between an MHC class II allele and clearance of hepatitis B virus in the Gambia. *New England Journal of Medicine* **332:** 1065–1069.

Tiwari JL & Terasaki PI (1985) *HLA and Disease Associations*, pp 232–263. New York: Springer-Verlag.

Todd JA & Bain SC (1992) A practical approach to identification of susceptibility genes for IDDM. *Diabetes* **41:** 1029–1034.

Todd JA, Bell JI & McDevitt HO (1987) HLA-DQβ gene contributes to susceptibility and resistance to insulin-dependent diabetes mellitus. *Nature* **329:** 599–604.

Underhill J, Donaldson P, Bray G et al (1992) Susceptibility to primary biliary cirrhosis is associated with the *HLA-DR8-DQB1*0402* haplotype. *Hepatology* **16:** 1404–1408.

Underhill JA, Donaldson PT, Doherty DG et al (1995) HLA DPB polymorphism in primary sclerosing cholangitis and primary biliary cirrhosis. *Hepatology* **21:** 959–962.

van Hattum J, Schreuder GM & Schalm SW (1987) HLA antigens in patients with various courses after hepatitis B virus infection. *Hepatology* **7:** 11–14.

Vergani D, Wells L, Larcher VF et al (1985) Genetically determined low C4: a predisposing factor to autoimmune chronic active hepatitis. *Lancet* **ii:** 294–298.

Weisman JY & Tsuchiyose MM (1988) Lack of a response to recombinant hepatitis B vaccine in non responders to plasma vaccine. *Journal of the American Medical Association* **260:** 1734–1738.

Williams DB & Watts TH (1995) Molecular chaperones in antigen presentation. *Current Opinion in Immunology* **7:** 77–84.

Index

Note: Page numbers of article titles are in **bold** type.

551